FUTURESCAN™ 2013

Healthcare Trends and Implications 2013–2018

CONTENTS

BETWEEN A ROCK AND A HARD PLACE

by Don Seymour

Healthcare is in a period of transition, one that arguably began with passage of the Accountable Care Act in 2010, as the volume-based payment model (the "first curve") gives way to a value-based model (the "second curve") (AHA 2011). Volume-based payment is rooted in the traditional, fee-for-service, acute care paradigm focused on illness—the one we all grew up with. The value-based payment model that is emerging focuses on quality, safety, patient satisfaction, and, of course, reduced cost. Providers will have to live "life in the gap" for the foreseeable future (Exhibit 0.1).

A menacing "third curve" also is emerging: a global payment model tied to population health management and focused on wellness, prevention, and management of chronic disease. It sounds good in public policy theory, but most of us have little to no experience with it. Life in the gap is one thing; life in the chasm will be far more challenging (Exhibit 0.1).

Perseverance, Ingenuity, and Fortitude

In 2004, Aron Ralston, a young mountaineer, published his autobiographical account of being trapped in Blue John Canyon in the Utah desert. When a falling boulder pinned his arm against the canyon wall, he was literally between a rock and a hard place, and this became the title of his autobiography (subsequently released as a movie titled *127 Hours*). The phrase originated in the early 1900s and is associated with the struggles of the mining and railroad industries in the western United States. It seems applicable, as well, to the challenge facing the nation's healthcare providers—systems, hospitals, and physicians in particular—as they struggle to stay alive in 2013, pinned between declining performance-based risk payment (the second curve) on one side and actuarial-based risk payment (the third curve) on the other. Mr. Ralston provides a metaphor for our struggle and an example of the perseverance, ingenuity, and fortitude that will be required for us to succeed.

Futurescan 2013 offers timely guidance from eight national experts on how we can survive our rock-and-a-hard-place and eventually walk out of the canyon. The excerpts below provide a glimpse into the insights awaiting the reader.

About the Author

Don Seymour, president of Don Seymour & Associates in Winchester, Massachusetts, has been a strategy adviser to hospital boards, chief executive officers, and medical staff leaders since 1979. A frequent presenter on subjects related to senior leadership in healthcare organizations, Seymour is on the faculty of the American College of Healthcare Executives and the Governance Institute. Additionally, he has made presentations to the American Hospital Association, numerous *Fortune 100* companies, and a variety of other national, state, and regional groups. He has served as executive editor of *Futurescan™* since 2004. A past president of the Society for Healthcare Strategy & Market Development, he received its Award for Individual Professional Excellence in 2008.

Exhibit 0.1 Changing Healthcare Payment Models

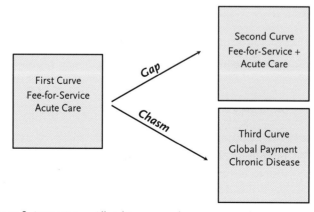

On insurer–provider integration:
Healthcare providers and insurers have before us a unique opportunity to collaborate … to design a delivery system that meets our respective business objectives while principally focusing on the patient. A central barrier to creating a healthcare system that provides Americans with the best, most affordable care possible is the high degree of fragmentation, [which] leads to uncoordinated care and misaligned incentives, driving up costs and too often distracting from what should be the paramount shared objective of all stakeholders: acting in the best interest of the patient who is seeking and getting care.—Scott P. Serota

On payment reform: From my perspective—touching data from hundreds of organizations across the healthcare spectrum—how organizations are responding to payment reform is more important than where they sit on the orthodox spectrum of integration, with fully integrated organizations (e.g., ACOs) on one end and the fragmented status quo on the other. In my view, the corporate form of a provider system will become a mostly irrelevant formal distinction—like the difference between HMOs and PPOs—rather than a mark of quality or efficiency.
—Bruce S. Pyenson

On nursing: Primary care in the United States is already struggling to meet patients' needs. [S]olutions must enable nurses, as well as other health professionals, to practice to the full extent of their education and training in a team-based model of care delivery. In many settings, advanced practice registered nurses … can be used to address the primary care staffing shortage and free up physicians to care for more complex cases requiring their expertise. Yet, many states have outdated regulations and barriers that prevent nurses from practicing to the

full extent of their education and training.—John W. Rowe, MD

On palliative care: Palliative care is specialized medical care for people with serious illnesses. This type of care focuses on providing patients with relief from symptoms, pain, and stress, whatever the diagnosis. Palliative medicine is a fast-growing medical specialty—palliative care programs are now in place at nearly 90 percent of large (>300 beds) US hospitals. It's no wonder why: Palliative care enhances patient and family satisfaction, improves quality, and can prolong survival, all at a fraction of the cost of "usual care." Studies demonstrate that palliative care programs can save hospitals millions of dollars per year.—Diane E. Meier, MD

On health information exchanges (HIEs): Hospital-based HIEs may prove to be the linchpin of future data exchange efforts by participating in whatever information exchanges—community, regional, or state-level—satisfy their clinical and financial business needs. By viewing data as a strategic lever, CEOs can position their organizations for long-term sustainability in the new era of payment reform; reduce expenses through avoidance of duplication and unnecessary procedures; and improve the quality of patient care and positive outcomes, thereby increasing patient satisfaction and engagement.—Carla Smith, John P. Hoyt, FACHE, and Pamela Matthews, RN

On mHealth: The new mobile paradigm requires a more consumer- and patient-oriented approach to medicine, one that uses mobile technology to increase feedback, change behaviors, and promote engagement and empowerment. By shifting power and control toward the patient, mHealth will change the fundamental nature of the provider–patient relationship. The changes facilitated by mobile

technology will enable providers to increase their productivity and efficiency, provide more frequent, lighter "touches" to more patients, and encourage a better approach to preventive healthcare and wellness. But such changes will also be painful and disruptive.—Christopher L. Wasden, EdD

On healthcare governance: Many boards have similar "DNA" passed down from hospital ancestors. They draw most trustees locally from the community's "elite" establishment, favoring individuals with business and finance backgrounds. Viewing board service as a volunteer position can lead to low expectations for participation. … Community boards so cherish local autonomy that they may not objectively evaluate strategic alliance and merger opportunities. The medical staff president and other officers may serve as ex officio representatives of a medical staff that is viewed not as a care partner, but warily as a semiautonomous entity with a self-centered economic agenda.—Barry S. Bader

On the Baldrige Criteria for Performance Excellence:
Managing a healthcare enterprise will become increasingly complex because of changes in regulation, consolidation, payment and reimbursement systems, uncertain economic conditions, and integrated delivery systems. To address these changes and the inherent uncertainty associated with them, leaders will have to be able to adjust strategy quickly and execute changes rapidly. Dealing with uncertainty by avoiding strategic planning will likely be fatal for an institution. Starting in 2013, the Baldrige Criteria will include a focus on dealing with strategy in uncertain times.—Harry S. Hertz, PhD, HFACHE

Leaving the Canyon

After several days alone, out of water and out of options to otherwise release himself, Mr. Ralston amputated his right arm and walked out of the canyon; he eventually returned to mountaineering. And that is the goal of *Futurescan*: to enable healthcare leaders to consider their options and find productive solutions (short of amputation!) to moving their organizations out of the canyon. You may not agree with all the assumptions our authors have made nor with their conclusions. We invited them to pen their pieces because we respect their expertise and believe they are right more often than not.

We also knew they would stimulate your thinking, and that ultimately is the purpose of *Futurescan*. More right than wrong? We certainly hope so, but, more important, we hope to have encouraged deeper thinking on important topics and provided leaders of the nation's hospitals and care delivery systems with a base of departure for discussion of eight critical leadership challenges. ▣

Reference

American Hospital Association (AHA). 2011. *Hospitals and Care Systems of the Future.* Report from the AHA Committee on Performance Improvement. Chicago: AHA.

1. INSURER–PROVIDER INTEGRATION

INSURERS AND PROVIDERS INTEGRATING TOWARD A COMMON CAUSE

by Scott P. Serota

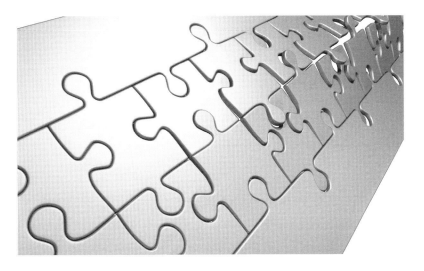

About the Author

Scott P. Serota is president and chief executive officer of the Blue Cross and Blue Shield Association (BCBSA), a national federation of 38 independent, community-based and locally operated Blue Cross and Blue Shield companies. He was named BCBSA president and CEO in 2000, after serving four years as a senior executive, including two years as chief operating officer. Before joining the Blues, Serota was president and CEO of Chicago-based Rush Prudential Health Plans, where he led the integration of Rush-Presbyterian-St. Luke's Medical Center Health Plans and The Prudential. Serota is a founding member of the National Business Group on Health's Institute on Healthcare Costs and Solutions and a board member of the Council for Affordable Quality Healthcare and of the Partnership for Prevention.

A central barrier to creating a healthcare system that provides Americans with the best, most affordable care possible is the high degree of fragmentation that traditionally has existed among the many parties involved in delivering, managing, financing, and receiving that care. Fragmentation leads to unco-ordinated care and misaligned incentives, which drive up costs and too often distract from what should be the paramount shared objective of all stakeholders: acting in the best interest of the patient who is seeking and getting care.

By contrast, greater integration among stakeholders—especially between healthcare providers and insurers—can serve to align incentives and create important efficiencies that engender more favorable results. As new payment approaches and practice models have demonstrated in recent years, efforts that lead to better alignment and shared risk show much promise.

That said, the present interest in and hopes for integration on the part of policymakers, pundits, and healthcare experts alike have inevi-tably drawn comparisons to earlier attempts to better align providers and insurers. But unique factors in the current environment—including heightened public and regulatory scrutiny, the greater economic risk of *not* addressing costs, more engaged healthcare consumers, and technological advances that enable powerful insights—present impor-tant differences from the past and justify the high expectations for the current movement.

Environmental Drivers

Public and regulatory pressures. The Affordable Care Act (ACA) imposes substantial change on all healthcare stakeholders, which in turn has cast a public spotlight on issues previously relegated mostly to thoughtful consideration by actuaries, academics, and policy practitioners.

For insurers, heightened public attention only reinforces our focus on managing medical and administrative costs and seeking higher-quality care in exchange for payments to provid-ers. Increased competition from the ACA-mandated health insurance exchanges, along with insurance reform provisions—such as guar-anteed issue, community rating, and medical-loss-ratio thresholds (Commonwealth Fund 2010)—are precipitating insurers' creation of new provider payment models, including much more collaborative risk-sharing relationships.

The ACA also holds hospitals and physicians more accountable for the quality of care they deliver, with community needs assessments, participation in quality transparency

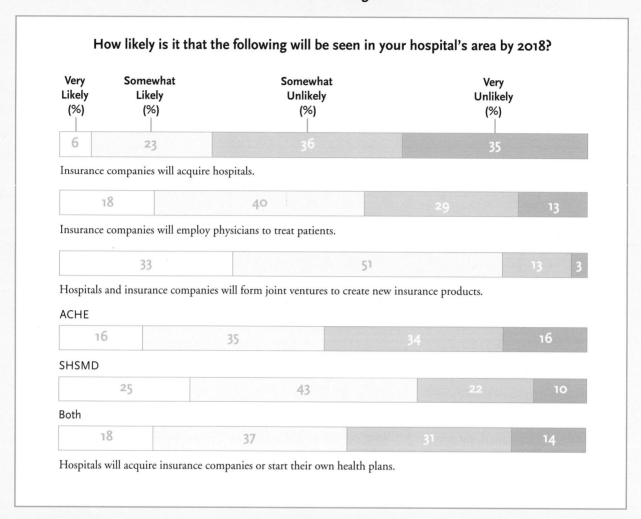

Note: Percentages in each row may not sum exactly to 100% due to rounding.

What Practitioners Predict

Hospitals and insurance companies will collaborate. Eighty-four percent of practitioners agreed that by 2018, hospitals and insurance companies will form joint ventures to create new insurance products.

Insurance companies are unlikely to acquire hospitals. Most practitioners were doubtful that insurance companies will acquire hospitals, with 71 percent of respondents indicating this as unlikely.

Opinions about other types of hospital–insurer relationships are mixed. A small majority (58 percent) said it is likely insurance companies will hire physicians to treat patients, and 55 percent said it is likely hospitals will acquire insurance companies or start their own health plans.

reporting initiatives, and greater involvement in fraud and abuse detection all outlined in the law's provisions (Commonwealth Fund 2010). Providers are looking to insurers for the expertise and data they need to adapt to these changes.

Market cost pressures. As they have for years, healthcare costs continue to outstrip general inflation rates. Even with lower utilization, which is widely believed to have been suppressed by American consumers' continuing economic struggles, health spending in 2010 rose by 3.9 percent (CMS 2011), a smaller increase than in the years before the recession but still above the average growth in consumer prices. The projection is for continued growth in health spending in 2013 and beyond. Moreover, given the struggling US economy, the country's worsening debt position, and the fact that healthcare now is responsible for nearly 18 percent of the gross domestic product (Council of Economic Advisers 2009), most everyone agrees these trends are simply unsustainable.

Consumerism. As healthcare costs continue to rise and as ACA provisions are phased in, consumers are being given greater responsibility for their health and healthcare decision making. As a result, consumers—who, through employer-sponsored coverage, traditionally have been largely shielded from the real costs of care—now face a myriad of decisions and, importantly, the bills resulting from those decisions. This trend is driving demand for more information and new solutions that will help consumers understand medical conditions, evaluate prescribed treatments and procedures, discern alternatives, and assess relative value for their healthcare dollar. These activities affect insurers and providers alike and so are driving both parties to collaborate to better serve the customer.

Data: the great enabler. Better coordinated care requires careful longitudinal tracking and objective assessment of that care, which in turn require a wealth of data. Rich sources of data—including providers' clinical patient records and insurers' administrative claims—remain largely untapped. But through electronic record keeping, faster data processing, and sophisticated analytic techniques, insurers and their provider partners today can uncover actionable insights to better understand and influence care.

An Evolving Definition

Facing these realities, healthcare insurers and providers have sought to bring their businesses closer together, leveraging the unique, complementary areas of expertise each brings to address the challenges that come with current industry dynamics. No doubt integration can be beneficial, to the degree it serves as a means to a shared end-goal: higher quality and more affordable healthcare.

Although integration is perhaps most commonly associated with vertical integrated delivery, in which insurers and hospital systems or provider groups are part of a single entity, in practice far more efforts have taken the form of aligned payment arrangements and structural collaboration toward new shared-responsibility practice models.

The following examples summarize three models of alignment present in the current market environment.

Pay-for-value, not volume. New reimbursement arrangements can better align financial incentives between health plans and providers. These payment strategies are moving the industry from fee-for-service and capitation models that lack quality requirements or efficiency standards to value-based models that reward provider coordination and improvements in quality processes and outcomes as well as efficiency. Blue Cross and Blue Shield pay-for-performance and episode-based payment strategies—now in place in nearly every state—have yielded hundreds of millions in savings, as well as material improvements in quality and patient safety.

Aligned practice. To support providers that accept greater risk and accountability, health plans are employing multiple payment strategies and structuring networks that reinforce primary care, enable total population management, and drive greater coordination across providers. Examples include patient-centered medical homes (PCMHs), which provide incentives for primary care providers to coordinate patients' care needs, and accountable care organizations (ACOs), in which a group of healthcare providers agrees to deliver coordinated care and meet performance benchmarks for quality and affordability to manage the total cost of care for its member population. PCMHs and ACOs involving Blue Cross and Blue Shield companies from California to New Jersey have achieved double-digit reductions in hospital admission rates, fewer ER visits, and lower overall medical costs (Blue Cross and Blue Shield Association 2012).

Joint ownership. In certain circumstances, insurers and providers seek a different level of integration to meet specific strategic objectives, such as diversifying revenue streams, creating efficiencies in serving high-cost segments, and hedging against physician shortages. For instance, a venture between Blue Cross and Blue Shield of North Carolina and the UNC Health Care System created a primary care physician practice to manage members' chronic conditions (Blue Cross and Blue Shield of North Carolina 2011). The model includes a multidisciplinary team of physicians, nurses, nutritionists, pharmacists, and behavioral health specialists.

Looking Ahead

Insurers and providers pursue each of these types of alignment for specific purposes in unique circumstances, and it is important to note that greater structural alignment does not necessarily equate to greater effectiveness. In this respect—and as the survey data collected for this report bear out—there is no discernible consensus that larger-scale structural models, such as acquisitions by insurers or providers, will dominate going forward.

What *is* now widely accepted is that our healthcare system needs to continue to move away from fee-for-service medicine, which puts incentives for providers into conflict with incentives for insurers.

As a result, aligned payment strategies will continue to evolve and become more pervasive in all markets. More formal collaborative solutions, such as ACOs and PCMHs, also will expand in scope and scale, as insurers increasingly see the need to give providers the administrative, technical, and clinical support they need to fully realize the potential of payment models. Under certain scenarios, additional hospital systems and insurers may align more closely through joint ventures, mergers, or acquisitions that approach or achieve more integrated delivery.

In short, observed and new forms of integration will continue as long as demands exist for higher-quality and lower-cost care. Insurers and providers each bring specialized expertise to address these demands—expertise that is better leveraged than duplicated in the current environment of increased cost pressure.

Implications for Hospital Leaders

Greater accountability will require hospital systems to manage risk by tracking patients throughout the entire care experience. By accepting greater financial risk for patients, hospitals transcend their traditional core competencies, making partnerships with health plans all the more important. Insurers can offer several complementary competencies—risk management, of course, but also a wealth of data and specialized health informatics skills with which to track and assess patients across the continuum of care in real time, not just the portion(s) provided directly by the hospital system.

Consumerism will continue to exert financial pressures, requiring hospitals to reconsider pricing and the roles they want to play. Educated and informed healthcare consumers will seek out and demand higher-quality care and better provider experiences. Facing more of the cost of care themselves, they will not tolerate confusing billing based on chargemasters or procedures that are priced substantially higher than those performed in other care settings. With declining margins, hospitals will need to carefully assess their competitive strengths and weaknesses and refocus their business strategy around activities that deliver the greatest value—that is, care that is most appropriately delivered at their facilities.

Public and government scrutiny will lead hospitals to assume a broader community role. Despite taking on greater risk amid financial constraints, hospitals will be expected to take on responsibility for the care delivered not just within their four walls, but also across the local communities they serve. Having received public funding for capital construction (and often favorable tax treatment as well), hospitals will be under increasing pressure to use high-cost assets for more than just traditional acute care services. Hospitals will be urged to take a more active role in improving the health status of the local population through greater outreach to the community and targeted patient education. Hospitals also will need to focus on educating new healthcare professionals to ensure that the communities they serve have a sufficient supply of caregivers.

Transparency and continued downward pressure on Medicare and Medicaid rates will require hospitals to become more efficient. The practice of protecting margins by shifting costs from publicly supported patients to commercially insured ones will become untenable as the components of price become more transparent and as patients increasingly compare costs—and outcome statistics—across hospitals (Proebsting 2010). Hospitals will need to tighten their cost structures while seeking new sources of revenue to maximize appropriate use of their existing infrastructure. ⬛

References

Blue Cross and Blue Shield Association. 2012. "Transforming Care Delivery: Care Delivery Programs Overview." Proprietary information released April 2.

Blue Cross and Blue Shield of North Carolina. 2011. "BCBSNC and UNC Health Care Open Carolina Advanced Health." News release issued December 7. www.bcbsnc.com/content/providers/news-and-information/news/dec7a-2011.htm.

Centers for Medicare & Medicaid Services (CMS). 2011. "National Health Expenditure Projections 2011–2021." Accessed August 16, 2012. www.cms.gov/research-statistics-data-and-systems/statistics-trends-and-reports/national healthexpenddata/downloads/proj2011pdf.pdf.

Commonwealth Fund. 2010. "Major Provisions of the Affordable Care Act." Published August 16. www.common wealthfund.org/~/media/files/publications/other/2010/timeline%20coverage_040110_v4.pdf.

Council of Economic Advisers. 2009. *The Economic Case for Health Care Reform.* Published June 2009. www.white house.gov/assets/documents/CEA_Health_Care_Report.pdf.

Proebsting, D. 2010. "Why Hospital Cost Shifting Is No Longer a Viable Strategy." Milliman Healthcare Reform Briefing Paper published June 24. http://insight.milliman.com/article.php?cntid=7254&utm_medium=web&utm_content=7254&utm_campaign=Milliman%20On%20Healthcare.

THE CALCULATED RISK OF PAYMENT REFORM

by Bruce S. Pyenson

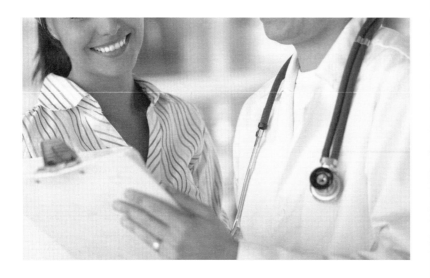

About the Author

Bruce S. Pyenson is a principal and consulting actuary in the New York office of Milliman, Inc., where his clients include healthcare businesses, integrated delivery systems, employers, providers, advocacy groups, HMOs, and biotechnology companies. Most of his projects involve integrating analytics from financial, clinical, and operational models to address issues ranging from market strategies and capitation to healthcare reform. In recent years, client projects have included assessment of pandemic influenza and lung cancer screening and mortality, healthcare reform evaluations for advocacy groups, and feasibility analyses for accountable care organizations. Pyenson is active in the C-Change cancer collaborative, and he serves on the board of The Health Project's Koop Awards. He is a Fellow of the Society of Actuaries and a member of the American Academy of Actuaries.

Political columnists are interpreting early results of accountable care organizations (ACOs) to bolster their opinions of healthcare reform (e.g., Pipes 2012). From my perspective—touching data from hundreds of organizations across the healthcare spectrum—how organizations are responding to payment reform is more important than where they sit on the orthodox spectrum of integration, with fully integrated organizations (e.g., ACOs) on one end and the fragmented status quo on the other. In my view, the corporate form of a provider system will become a mostly irrelevant formal distinction—like the difference between HMOs and PPOs—rather than a mark of quality or efficiency.

Payment reform should be viewed in the context of increasing financial and market pressures. With the weak economy and healthcare reform, the fundamentals of finance have changed. Consumer expectations also have changed; they are set by iPhones and Droids rather than by our grandfathers' post office. Some of our hospital clients expect all contracts to be performance based within a few years.

In the new payment environment, I expect the winners will be organizations that can quickly adapt to change. This is a better predictor of success than organizations' embracing one or another tactic.

Health Insurers: Examples of Quick Change to Payment Reform

The speed of changes accomplished by the health insurance industry serves as an impressive example to hospitals. In a few short years, many "business as usual" practices that existed for decades, such as limits on coverage for preexisting conditions, medical underwriting, and annual and lifetime limits, have been or will soon be abandoned. Likewise, many new policies have been implemented, such as minimum loss ratios, rate approvals, changes to financial reporting, coverage for adult children, preventive services with no cost sharing, and changes to premium rate structures. Insurers are actively preparing to participate in health insurance exchanges in 2014, although whether particular insurers will participate will depend on the yet-to-be-released rules. The Affordable Care Act (ACA) set a schedule for the changes; the alternative for insurers was to stop insuring health.

Hospitals far outnumber insurers (6,000 versus 600), and certainly some venerable health insurers' exit from the health business (e.g., The Principal) coincided with healthcare reform. At the same time, a number of new insurance start-ups, some funded by venture capital and others funded by provider groups, are looking at the new models proposed by healthcare reform as business opportunities.

The ACA seems to have been gentler to non-insurers in healthcare—so far. The pharmaceutical industry has certainly faced changes—more discounts to Medicaid, transparency in dealing with physicians, and new approval processes for biological drugs. Hospitals face penalties from Medicare for readmissions, and Medicare seems to be slowly adopting private-insurer techniques, independently of healthcare reform. Some of the changes to date have been carrots rather than sticks. Of special relevance to our discussion are opportunities from the Centers for Medicare & Medicaid Services, including

- ACOs, such as the Medicare Shared Savings Program (MSSP) and the Pioneer ACO model, and
- the Bundled Payment for Care Improvement Initiative (BPCII).

My experience since the 1990s working with organizations that are considering ACOs and bundled payments have led me to reject the usual "spectrum of integration" distinction in favor of a "culture of change" characterization.

Payment Reform Means Less Payment

According to the *Futurescan* survey, most respondents expect inpatient admissions to decrease. I agree and would like to offer some insight into the underlying dynamics.

Healthcare-acquired infections, readmissions, and ambulatory care–sensitive admissions will decrease. These issues are the

three "bad boys" of admissions and markers of quality problems. But a recent *Health Affairs* article shows that better care does not reduce cost significantly, at least for diabetes (Eddy and Shah 2012). Furthermore, my colleagues have observed that readmission rates parallel admission rates—in other words, organizations that have lower admission rates also have lower readmission rates. Finally, ambulatory care–sensitive admissions are a fairly constant percentage of total admission rates. Many regions have a lot of medically unnecessary admissions. The bottom line: If you succeed at reducing these bad boys, a lot of other admissions will go away, too.

Elective procedures will decrease as patient cost sharing increases. The ACA sets the coverage percentages (really the actuarial value) of exchange plans at 90 percent (Platinum), 80 percent (Gold), 70 percent (Silver), and 60 percent (Bronze). These levels establish a new standard for insurance and benefits. Although most people would consider the Silver and Bronze levels to be rather poor coverage, insurers are already downshifting benefits to conform to these new, lower standards and prevent adverse selection. A new name for elective procedures is "preference sensitive"; patients selecting the new, lower coverage levels are likely to choose treatments with lower out-of-pocket costs.

Hospitals and insurance companies will form joint ventures to create new insurance products. The exchange marketplace will allow individuals to shop for their insurance and pay for their choice. As a hypothetical example, "Community Hospital ACO" co-marketed with an insurer could be low priced because it restricts care to a limited network. Such products might become as successful as similar low-priced, limited-

network products sold to seniors in Medicare Part D. They will succeed to the extent that they reduce healthcare spending.

The *Futurescan* survey results seem credible given that forces from healthcare reform, payers, the economy, and consumers all are pushing in the same direction.

A Spectrum of Responses to Payment Reform Opportunities

Organizations considering the new opportunities can respond either traditionally or more expansively (Exhibit 2.1). In my experience, more advanced organizations continue to take the traditional approach to evaluation but also bring a broader perspective.

Some potential bundled-payment applicants taking the traditional approach to evaluation rejected the BPCII when they saw the required discount to Medicare as a loss of income; they could not assess the potential upside of controlling post-acute care or the value of bonding with their physicians. Several other hospitals rejected bundled payments for hip and knee arthroplasty because their affiliated orthopedic surgeons had little knowledge about what happens to their patients in the 30 or 60 days following discharge and could not assess the available data. These organizations could not transcend the traditional approach, which usually means comparing next year's fees to last year's fees.

The most sophisticated organizations also start by comparing a proposal with the status quo. But they know the status quo may be disappearing, so they compare the proposal with other alternatives as well. For example, one hospital system declined to apply to the Medicare ACO program because it could get a better deal through its affiliated Medicare Advantage

Evaluation Approach	Organizations Using Traditional Evaluation (less advanced)	Organizations Using System Change Evaluation (more advanced) = Likely Winners
The opportunity is like a managed care negotiation. Compare revenue to current fee-for-service levels. How much revenue will we lose?	X	X
The opportunity is a learning experience. How much will it cost to learn?		X
The opportunity has pros and cons. What are the advantages relative to other current and future opportunities?		X

plan. Another organization, a Pioneer ACO, declined to apply for bundled payments because many of those cases were already included among the lives attributed to the ACO. Both organizations had also compared MSSP or BPCII with the fee-for-service status quo, but they didn't stop there.

Although all the examples above led to a "reject the offer" decision, the differences in the hospitals' use of data and depth of thinking are more striking than the different decisions they made.

Runners and Walkers, but Not Many Joggers

BPCII has often been presented as "ACO lite" for hospitals interested in ACOs but not yet ready for the more comprehensive MSSP or the Pioneer ACO model. However, the tepid response suggests that surprisingly few hospitals are seeking a moderate-risk path. In other words, although leading organizations are willing to take bigger risks for bigger rewards, such as Medicare shared savings, for many others the effort to make bundled payments work does not seem balanced by the potential reward. The biggest groups seem to be the runners and the walkers, not the joggers in between.

The Demand for Payment Reform Talent

Futurescan survey respondents overwhelmingly believe health information exchanges and mHealth (mobile health) technology will be part of their future over the next five years. Although I agree that these developments will be basic infrastructural requirements for business, the capacity of an organization's management, board, and physicians to respond to payment reform depends on human capital. Leading organizations display the following characteristics:

- Leaders who survived the "PHO (physician–hospital organization) wars" of the 1990s with open minds (and probably some scars!)
- Decades of experience with alternative forms of reimbursement
- Senior staff who have worked in, and could return to, the insurance industry
- Finance staff who are an integral part of risk assessment

- Medical leadership that appreciates how administrative excellence can promote excellent outcomes

A major factor limiting the pace of change will be a shortage of "new era" leaders and talent at the executive, operational, finance, and clinical levels. To succeed at payment reform, a hospital needs a depth of financial, network, medical, and administrative talent. Many hospitals have been quietly building their talent pools for years, with or without formal ACO organizations. There are definitely some "sleeper" organizations waiting for the right opportunity.

Implications for Hospital Leaders

Hospital organizations that respond to opportunities strategically will have significant leverage in dealing with insurers. There are a few hundred such organizations across the United States. That rough figure is based on the number of hospitals participating in various leadership and industry organizations and applicants for the Medicare Shared

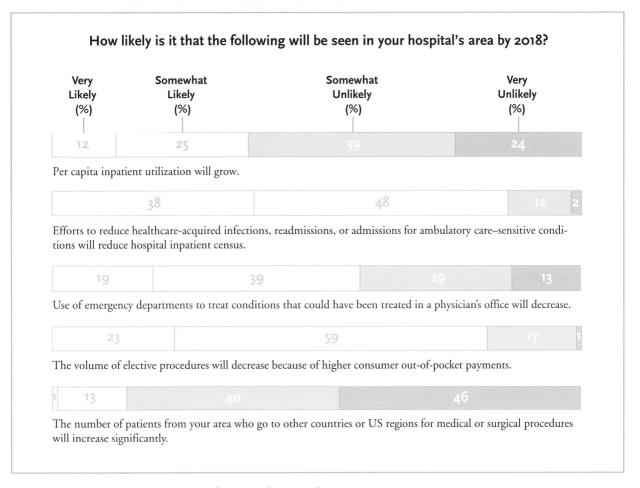

How likely is it that the following will be seen in your hospital's area by 2018?

Very Likely (%)	Somewhat Likely (%)	Somewhat Unlikely (%)	Very Unlikely (%)
12	25	39	24

Per capita inpatient utilization will grow.

38	48	12	2

Efforts to reduce healthcare-acquired infections, readmissions, or admissions for ambulatory care–sensitive conditions will reduce hospital inpatient census.

19	39	29	13

Use of emergency departments to treat conditions that could have been treated in a physician's office will decrease.

23	59	17	1

The volume of elective procedures will decrease because of higher consumer out-of-pocket payments.

1	13	40	46

The number of patients from your area who go to other countries or US regions for medical or surgical procedures will increase significantly.

Note: Percentages in each row may not sum exactly to 100% due to rounding.

What Practitioners Predict

Hospital inpatient census will be reduced because of hospital efforts. Eighty-six percent of practitioners agreed that by 2018 hospital inpatient censuses will have been reduced through hospital efforts to reduce healthcare-acquired infections, hospital readmissions, and admissions for ambulatory care–sensitive conditions.

The volume of elective procedures will decrease. According to 82 percent of practitioners, the volume of elective procedures will decrease by 2018 because of higher consumer out-of-pocket expenses.

Medical tourism is not likely to increase. Most practitioners (86 percent) thought it unlikely that medical tourism will increase significantly by 2018.

Predictions are mixed about other aspects of utilization. There was less consensus about how other aspects of utilization might change by 2018. A small majority of practitioners (63 percent) did not think per capita inpatient utilization would grow, and nearly 58 percent predicted a decrease in the use of emergency departments to treat conditions that could have been treated in a physician's office.

Savings Program, as well as the fact that it's such hard work to create all the competencies needed to run an ACO. The top 10 percent will be the "haves."

A second tier of hospital organizations will participate in payer-sponsored ACOs while continuing with fee-for-service business. They will be characterized as lower-cost, local alternatives. In some locales, these organizations will consolidate as inpatient utilization decreases.

A small group of well-capitalized academic medical centers will continue with their missions. They will, however, make some adaptations to the new environment.

New organizations will emerge to fill newly discovered, unmet needs as the system consolidates. These organizations may specialize in managed care for dual eligibles (Medicare and Medicaid), post-acute care, or transitions in care.

The majority of payer contracts with hospitals will contain performance-based compensation within five years. Even in markets with open networks (e.g., PPOs), payers will attribute lives to particular systems and hold providers accountable for results.

Disclaimer

The opinions expressed in this article are those of the author and not necessarily those of Milliman, Inc. ⒡⒮

References

Eddy, D.M., and R. Shah. 2012. "A Simulation Shows Limited Savings from Meeting Quality Targets Under the Medicare Shared Savings Program." *Health Affairs* 31 (11): 1–9.

Pipes, S. 2012. "Forget About Providers, What Do Doctors Think of Obamacare?" *Forbes*. Published September 17. www.forbes.com/sites/sallypipes/2012/09/17/forget-about-providers-what-do-doctors-think-of-obamacare/.

3. NURSING TRANSITIONS IN NURSING PRESENT CHALLENGES AND OPPORTUNITIES FOR HOSPITALS

by John W. Rowe, MD

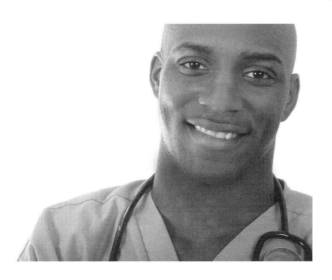

About the Author

John W. Rowe, MD, is a professor in the Department of Health Policy and Management at the Columbia University Mailman School of Public Health in New York City. From 2000 until late 2006, Dr. Rowe served as chairman and chief executive officer of Aetna, Inc., one of the nation's leading healthcare benefits organizations. From 1998 to 2000, he served as president and chief executive officer of Mount Sinai–NYU Health, one of the nation's largest academic healthcare organizations. Before joining Mount Sinai, Dr. Rowe was a professor of medicine and the founding director of the Division on Aging at the Harvard Medical School, as well as chief of gerontology at Boston's Beth Israel Hospital. He is an elected member of the Institute of Medicine and was a member of the committee that drafted *The Future of Nursing*.

Nursing, the largest segment of the US healthcare workforce, is in transition. As the era of accountable care organizations (ACOs) is ushered in and many provisions of the Affordable Care Act begin to be implemented, nurses can and should play a fundamental role in the transformation of the healthcare system. Hospital leaders need to understand how changes in nursing can enhance the likelihood that their hospitals will succeed in an increasingly competitive and financially difficult environment.

A convenient starting point for consideration of current trends in nursing is the landmark 2011 report *The Future of Nursing*, released by the Institute of Medicine (IOM 2011) in collaboration with the Robert Wood Johnson Foundation (RWJF). That report attracted wide attention, and AARP and RWJF have spearheaded an ambitious national campaign to implement the report's recommendations. To date, more than 80 organizations have joined this effort (Center to Champion Nursing in America 2012).

Let's review the implications of several of the IOM report's recommendations for hospital leaders.

IOM Recommendation: Remove Scope-of-Practice Barriers

Primary care in the United States is already struggling to meet patients' needs, and staffing shortages will only be exacerbated over the next decade as millions of newly insured Americans seek care and the population continues to age. For both immediate and long-term needs, solutions must enable nurses, as well as other health professionals, to practice to the full extent of their education and training in a team-based model of care delivery. In many settings, advanced practice registered nurses, who have been shown to provide general primary care that is as effective and safe as that delivered by physicians (Newhouse et al. 2011), can be used to address the primary care staffing shortage and free up physicians to care for more complex cases requiring their expertise.

Yet, many states have outdated regulations and barriers that prevent nurses from practicing to the full extent of their education and training. Although some states allow nurse practitioners to see patients and prescribe medications without a physician's supervision, a majority of states do not (AANP 2011). The variability of scope-of-practice regulations across states may hinder nurse practitioners from managing the care they were trained to provide and contributing to innovative healthcare delivery solutions.

Currently 16 states permit nurses to diagnose and treat patients independent of direct physician supervision, and the issue is under consideration in many states that currently restrict such scope of nursing practice.

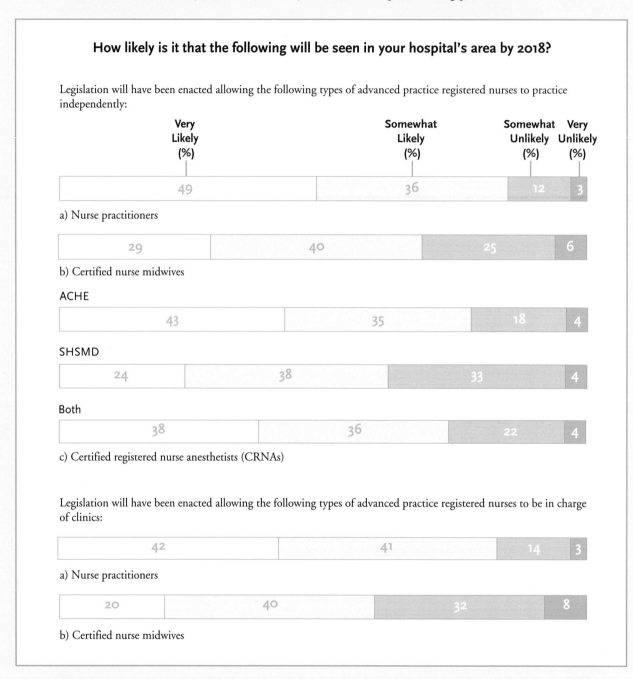

How likely is it that the following will be seen in your hospital's area by 2018?

Legislation will have been enacted allowing the following types of advanced practice registered nurses to practice independently:

	Very Likely (%)	Somewhat Likely (%)	Somewhat Unlikely (%)	Very Unlikely (%)
	49	36	12	3

a) Nurse practitioners

	29	40	25	6

b) Certified nurse midwives

ACHE

	43	35	18	4

SHSMD

	24	38	33	4

Both

	38	36	22	4

c) Certified registered nurse anesthetists (CRNAs)

Legislation will have been enacted allowing the following types of advanced practice registered nurses to be in charge of clinics:

	42	41	14	3

a) Nurse practitioners

	20	40	32	8

b) Certified nurse midwives

Note: Percentages in each row may not sum exactly to 100% due to rounding.

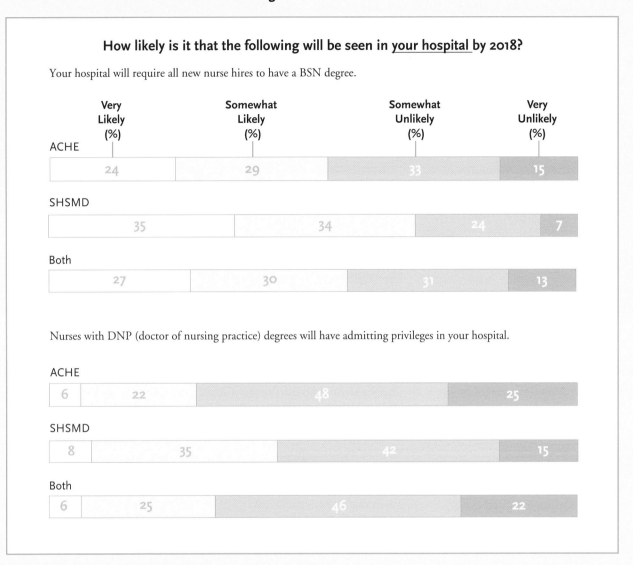

How likely is it that the following will be seen in <u>your hospital</u> by 2018?

Your hospital will require all new nurse hires to have a BSN degree.

	Very Likely (%)	Somewhat Likely (%)	Somewhat Unlikely (%)	Very Unlikely (%)
ACHE	24	29	33	15
SHSMD	35	34	24	7
Both	27	30	31	13

Nurses with DNP (doctor of nursing practice) degrees will have admitting privileges in your hospital.

	Very Likely (%)	Somewhat Likely (%)	Somewhat Unlikely (%)	Very Unlikely (%)
ACHE	6	22	48	25
SHSMD	8	35	42	15
Both	6	25	46	22

Note: Percentages in each row may not sum exactly to 100% due to rounding.

What Practitioners Predict

The scope of responsibilities for nurse practitioners and CRNAs will increase. Eighty-five percent of practitioners surveyed predict that by 2018 nurse practitioners will be able to practice independently, and 83 percent believe they will be allowed to be in charge of clinics. Seventy-four percent of practitioners believe CRNAs will be able to practice independently.

Results are more mixed with respect to responsibilities of certified nurse midwives. A smaller majority of practitioners (69 percent) predict that certified nurse midwives will be able to practice independently by 2018, and 60 percent believe they will be allowed to run clinics.

Results are mixed about admitting privileges for nurses with DNP (doctor of nursing practice) degrees and about requiring BSN degrees for new nurse hires. Practitioners surveyed were skeptical that nurses with DNP degrees would have admitting privileges at their hospitals by 2018, with more than 68 percent saying this was unlikely. Practitioners were more equally split on whether their hospitals would require nurses to have BSN degrees as a condition of hire by 2018, with 57 percent indicating this as likely.

IOM Recommendation: Increase the Proportion of Nurses with a Bachelor's Degree to 80 Percent by 2020

Hospitals have good reasons to hire more nurses who have a bachelor of science in nursing (BSN). As the federal government implements pay-for-performance changes in the next couple of years, hospitals will need well-trained healthcare professionals who can manage complex situations and quickly adapt to new roles. They will need employees who work well in teams and can recognize areas where improvements can be made. Several studies support a significant association between the educational level of registered nurses and outcomes for patients in the acute care setting, including mortality rates (Aiken et al. 2003; Estabrooks et al. 2005; Friese et al. 2008; Tourangeau et al. 2007; Van den Heede et al. 2009). Hospitals will need employees who can leverage critical thinking skills to solve complex problems and interact with appropriate technology to achieve efficiency and quality. BSN-prepared nurses are more likely than nurses with associate's degrees to be able to fill these roles.

BSN-prepared nurses are also more likely to be able to take on increasingly complex roles to improve organizational performance. They can serve as "nurse navigators," helping patients understand care options, insurance rules, and the healthcare system in general. Nurses who are trained in the best practices of care coordination can effectively manage patients in and between different healthcare settings and could help to prevent expensive disruptions in the delivery of care. This model would particularly benefit hospitals participating in ACOs.

Magnet status, often believed to distinguish a hospital in the marketplace, is another reason hospitals should hire more BSN-prepared nurses. The Magnet Recognition Program of the American Nurses Credentialing Center recognizes healthcare organizations for high-quality patient care, nursing excellence, and innovations in professional nursing practice. Starting in 2013, all nurse managers and nurse leaders in healthcare organizations seeking Magnet recognition will be required to have at least a BSN at the time the organization applies for Magnet status (ANCC 2012b). Furthermore, the Magnet program announced in 2012 that both current Magnet hospitals and all new applicants will need to submit a plan for achieving a nursing workforce that is 80 percent BSN prepared by 2020 (ANCC 2012a). Right now, far too few nurses continue with their education despite a desire to do so. Some of the hurdles they face are financial; others stem from the need to balance work schedules with family commitments.

IOM Recommendation: Expand Opportunities for Nurses to Lead and Diffuse Collaborative Improvement Efforts

Nurses bring an important voice and point of view to management and policy discussions. More nurses need to be prepared to lead improvement efforts in healthcare quality, safety, access, and value. And leadership needs to happen at every level.

Effective coordination and communication among health professionals can enhance the quality and safety of patient care. Physicians, nurses, pharmacists, and others who work collaboratively as integrated teams draw on individual and collective skills and experience across disciplines. They seek input and respect the contributions of everyone involved, empowering each team member to practice at a higher level. The inevitable result is better patient outcomes, including higher levels of patient satisfaction.

IOM Recommendation: Implement Nurse Residency Programs

Nurse residency programs—planned periods during which nursing graduates can acquire the knowledge and skills they need to deliver safe, high quality patient care—have been shown to significantly reduce turnover of new nursing staff (Goode et al. 2009; Krozek 2008). By reducing turnover, nurse residency programs both improve quality of care and lower much of the cost associated with the all-too-common "churn" among recent nursing grads introduced to the highly complex and stressful inpatient environment of a modern US hospital.

IOM Recommendation: Diversify the Healthcare Workforce

Finally, the IOM report and the AARP–RWJF campaign aim to diversify the healthcare workforce. Approximately 33 percent of the US population is part of a racial or ethnic minority group (US Census Bureau 2008), yet only 18 percent of nursing students are underrepresented minorities (Grumbach and Mendoza 2008). By 2050, African Americans, Asians, Latinos, and American Indians / Alaska Natives will account for a majority of the US population (US Census Bureau 2008).

Implications for Hospital Leaders

Allow nurses to practice at the top of their licenses. To respond effectively to the increased demand for primary care and innovative, interdisciplinary models of care, hospitals must be in a position to maximize the contributions of their nursing staffs. In states where scope-of-practice rules are restrictive, hospital leaders should support initiatives to permit nurses to practice independently to the full extent of their competence and certification.

The use of nurses to the fullest extent of their education and training is exemplified by the clinical nurse leader (CNL) model. CNLs are MSN-prepared nurses accountable for the healthcare outcomes of a specific group of patients within a unit or setting (AACN 2007). CNLs design, implement, and evaluate client care by coordinating, delegating, and supervising the care provided by the healthcare team, which includes licensed nurses, technicians, and other health professionals. The CNL model can be used to promote evidence-based medicine and improve patient quality.

Require newly hired nurses to have a BSN or to enroll in a BSN program. The most effective way to increase the number of BSN-prepared nurses is for hospitals to require that nurses complete a BSN program, as North Shore–LIJ Health System did (2010). Hospital leaders can hire more BSN-prepared nurses, or they can encourage nurses with associate's degrees to enter BSN programs within a specified time by offering tuition reimbursement, sala-ry differential, and promotion opportunities and by creating a culture that fosters continuing education through practices such as flextime.

Hospitals must form strong partnerships to achieve an 80 percent BSN-prepared workforce by 2020. Practice environments that support and enhance professional competence are essential to improving care. Hospitals should work with nursing schools to design and implement simulation labs and clinical training settings so that more BSN students can be educated simultaneously and gain clinical experience.

Financial assistance is available for this purpose from RWJF, which is establishing Academic Progression in Nursing programs in nine states (RWJF 2012). These states will receive funding of up to $300,000 over two years and will be looking to partner with healthcare facilities to implement one of four promising models promoting academic progression.

Encourage leadership opportunities for nurses. Hospital leaders should enable nurses to take the lead in developing and adopting innovative, patient-centered care models. They should encourage nurses and other frontline staff to work with developers and manufacturers in designing, developing, purchasing, implementing, and evaluating medical devices and health information technology.

Establish residency programs for new nurse graduates. Hospital leaders should fund the development and implementation of nurse residency programs across all practice settings. Hospitals that already offer nurse residency programs should evaluate their effectiveness in improving nurse retention, expanding competencies, and improving patient outcomes.

Seek to increase diversity. Hospital leaders need to make sure that the nursing profession reflects the diversity of the patients it serves and that all nurses deliver culturally competent care. Commitment to this goal and aggressive action by hospital leaders can have a dramatic effect on the recruitment of a diverse healthcare workforce.

Conclusion

If the US healthcare system is to meet the challenges of providing high-quality, cost-effective care while delivering primary care to millions of additional individuals, it must enhance the effectiveness of one of its critical and often neglected components—nursing. Hospitals can enhance their financial performance and competitiveness if they proactively embrace nursing reforms and advancements.

Acknowledgment

The author thanks Sue Hassmiller of the Robert Wood Johnson Foundation for her assistance in the preparation of this essay. ✍

References

Aiken, L.H., S.P. Clarke, R.B. Cheung, D.M. Sloane, and J.H. Silber. 2003. "Educational Levels of Hospital Nurses and Surgical Patient Mortality." *Journal of the American Medical Association* 290 (12): 1617–23.

American Academy of Nurse Practitioners (AANP). 2011. "Collaboration/Supervisory Language in State Practice Acts & Regulations for Nurse Practitioners." Updated August 9. www.aanp.org/images/documents/state-leg-reg/StateRegulatoryMap.pdf.

American Association of Colleges of Nursing (AACN). 2007. *White Paper on the Education and Role of the Clinical Nurse Leader*. Revised July 27. www.aacn.nche.edu/publications/white-papers/ClinicalNurseLeader.pdf.

American Nurses Credentialing Center (ANCC). 2012a. "Magnet Recognition Program FAQ: Data and Expected Outcomes." Updated July 27. www.nursecredentialing.org/Functional Category/FAQs/DEO-FAQ.aspx.

———. 2012b. "Organization Eligibility Requirements." Accessed September 25. www.nursecredentialing.org/OrgEligibilityRequirements.aspx.

Center to Champion Nursing in America. 2012. "Who's Involved." Accessed October 23. www.campaignforaction.org/whos-involved.

Estabrooks, C.A., W.K. Midodzi, G.G. Cummings, K.L. Ricker, and P. Giovanetti. 2005. "The Impact of Hospital Nursing Characteristics on 30-Day Mortality." *Nursing Research* 54 (2): 74–84.

Friese, C.R., E.T. Lake, L.H. Aiken, J.H. Silber, and J. Sochalski. 2008. "Hospital Nurse Practice Environments and Outcomes for Surgical Oncology Patients." *Health Services Research* 43 (4): 1145–63.

Goode, C.J., M.R. Lynn, C. Krsek, and G.D. Bednash. 2009. "Nurse Residency Programs: An Essential Requirement for Nursing." *Nursing Economics* 27 (3): 142–47, 159.

Grumbach, K., and R. Mendoza. 2008. "Disparities in Human Resources: Addressing the Lack of Diversity in the Health Professions." *Health Affairs* 27 (2): 413–22.

Institute of Medicine (IOM). 2011. *The Future of Nursing: Leading Change, Advancing Health*. Washington, DC: National Academies Press.

Krozek, C. 2008. "The New Graduate RN Residency: Win/Win/Win for Nurses, Hospitals, and Patients." *Nurse Leader* 6 (5): 41–44.

Newhouse, R.P., J. Stanik-Hutt, K.M. White, M. Johantgen, E.B. Bass, G. Zangaro, R.F. Wilson, L. Fountain, D.M. Steinwachs, L. Heindel, and J.P. Weiner. 2011. "Advanced Practice Nurse Outcomes 1990–2008: A Systematic Review." *Nursing Economics* 29 (5): 230–50.

North Shore–LIJ Health System. 2010. "North Shore–LIJ Becomes NY's First Health System to Require New Nurses to Get Bachelor's Degree." News release issued July 8. www.northshorelij.com/NSLIJ/New+Nurses+Required+to+Get+Bachelors+Degree.

Robert Wood Johnson Foundation (RWJF). 2012. "RWJF Launches New Initiative to Support Academic Progression in Nursing." News release issued March 22. www.rwjf.org/en/blogs/human-capital-blog/2012/03/rwjf-launches-new-initiative-to-support-academic-progression-in-nursing.html.

Tourangeau, A.E., D.M. Doran, L.M. Hall, L.O. Pallas, D. Pringle, J.V. Tu, and L.A. Cranley. 2007. "Impact of Hospital Nursing Care on 30-Day Mortality for Acute Medical Patients." *Journal of Advanced Nursing* 57 (1): 32–44.

US Census Bureau. 2008. "An Older and More Diverse Nation by Midcentury." News release issued August 14. www.census.gov/newsroom/releases/archives/population/cb08-123.html.

Van den Heede, K., E. Lesaffre, L. Diya, A. Vleugels, S.P. Clarke, L.H. Aiken, and W. Sermeus. 2009. "The Relationship Between Inpatient Cardiac Surgery Mortality and Nurse Numbers and Educational Level: Analysis of Administrative Data." *International Journal of Nursing Studies* 46 (6): 796–803.

4. PALLIATIVE CARE

BETTER CARE FOR THE SERIOUSLY ILL, BETTER VALUE FOR THE HEALTHCARE SYSTEM

by Diane E. Meier, MD

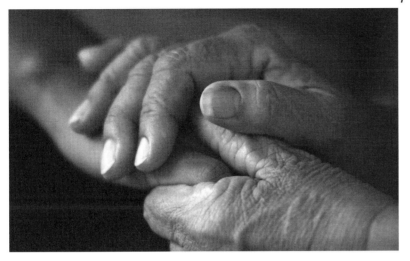

About the Author

Diane E. Meier, MD, is director of the Center to Advance Palliative Care, a national organization devoted to increasing the number and quality of palliative care programs in the United States. Under her leadership the number of palliative care programs in US hospitals has more than tripled in the past ten years. She is also the vice chair for public policy at the Hertzberg Palliative Care Institute and professor of geriatrics and internal medicine and Catherine Gaisman professor of medical ethics at Mount Sinai School of Medicine in New York City. Dr. Meier is the recipient of numerous awards, including the MacArthur Foundation Fellowship ("genius award") in 2008, the HealthLeaders 20 People Who Make Healthcare Better award (2010), the Alexander Richman Commemorative Award for Humanism in Medicine, the Founders Award of the National Hospice and Palliative Care Organization, AARP's 50th Anniversary Social Impact Award, and the American Academy of Hospice and Palliative Medicine Lifetime Achievement Award.

Palliative medicine is a fast-growing medical specialty—palliative care programs are now in place at nearly 90 percent of large (>300 beds) US hospitals (CAPC 2012). It's no wonder why: Palliative care enhances patient and family satisfaction, improves quality, and can prolong survival, all at a fraction of the cost of "usual care." Studies demonstrate that palliative care programs can save hospitals millions of dollars per year (Morrison et al. 2008).

Before reviewing the evidence for these claims and presenting a road map for the future, let's define palliative care accurately, given that there is sometimes confusion about how it differs from hospice (Exhibit 4.1).

Palliative Care Defined

Palliative care is specialized medical care for people with serious illnesses. This type of care focuses on providing patients with relief from symptoms, pain, and stress, whatever the diagnosis. The goal is to improve quality of life for both patients and their families. Palliative care is provided by a team of doctors, nurses, and other specialists who work with a patient's other doctors to provide an extra layer of support. Palliative care is appropriate at any age and at any stage of a serious illness and can be provided together with curative treatment.

In practice, interdisciplinary palliative care teams focus on relief of symptoms, including pain, fatigue, anxiety, and depression; expert communication with patients, families, and other health professionals about achievable goals of care and care plans to achieve those goals; and communication, continuity, and coordination of care across the many settings traversed by persons living with serious illness.

What Is the Relationship Between Hospice and Palliative Care?

Hospice is a form of palliative care that is limited to the dying. It is provided under a special Medicare benefit and is restricted to patients with a six-month prognosis who are willing to choose hospice care over curative or life-prolonging treatments. Because, under Medicare rules, patients may not receive hospice and disease treatment simultaneously, the median length of stay in hospice in the United States is only two to three weeks, and 30 percent of all hospice beneficiaries receive hospice care for less than a week (NHPCO 2012).

By contrast, palliative care teams serve patients based on need—independent of prognosis—whether

Exhibit 4.1 The Palliative Care–Hospice Care Spectrum

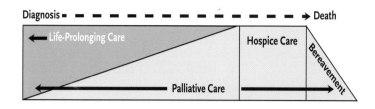

Source: Reprinted with permission from Adler et al. (2009).

the goal of care is cure (e.g., acute leukemia); life prolongation (e.g., heart failure, chronic lung disease); or ensuring peaceful and dignified care during a progressive illness, regardless of disease type (ideally provided in hospice for those who will clearly and predictably die within weeks to a few months).

Palliative care teams engage from diagnosis onward to minimize pain, nausea, and other symptoms; to preserve options and choices; to listen to and clarify the values and wishes of patients and their families and how those preferences relate to the care plan; and to improve communication among patient, family, and various specialists and sites of care. Unlike hospice patients, palliative care patients do not have to forgo treatment (e.g., a clinical trial or another course of chemotherapy) to receive the support and assistance of the palliative care team.

Growth of Palliative Care Services

The growth in the number of hospital palliative care teams in the past ten years has been nothing short of stunning. As of 2010, more than 65 percent of US hospitals with more than 50 beds reported having a palliative care team, including 88 percent of large (>300 bed) hospitals (CAPC 2012). In recognition of the impor-

tance of palliative care to hospital quality, The Joint Commission (2012) launched a new Advanced Certification Program for Palliative Care in 2011 for hospital inpatient programs that demonstrate exceptional patient- and family-centered care and optimize the quality of life for patients with serious illnesses.

Forces Driving the Adoption of Palliative Care

Palliative care improves quality. In the context of value-based purchasing, which links payment to quality outcomes, the imperative for hospitals and health systems to increase and sustain the highest levels of quality has never been greater. Although the highest-risk patients with serious illnesses, multimorbidity, and significant pain and symptoms typically represent only 5 to 10 percent of total admissions, they are disproportionately vulnerable to adverse events, such as hospital-acquired infections, pressure ulcers, medication errors, and rapid-cycle readmissions. Complicating management, these outliers are scattered throughout the health system.

Palliative care teams provide a "quarterback" support and coordination function, bringing expertise to care for complex, high-risk patients across all silos (specialties and inpatient units). Palliative care strengthens two areas that have long

been weak spots in US healthcare: It offers state-of-the-art techniques for managing pain and other symptoms, and it provides the time and expertise needed for long, often difficult patient and family meetings about prognosis, goals of care, and the patient's wishes and values. Numerous studies and meta-analyses have demonstrated that palliative care improves pain and symptom management, emotional and spiritual support, communication, and patient and family satisfaction (Bakitas et al. 2009; Meier 2011; Temel et al. 2010; Wright et al. 2008).

Concurrent palliative care may prolong survival. Researchers at Dana–Farber Cancer Institute conducted a randomized trial of palliative care with oncology comanagement for newly diagnosed lung cancer patients. The comanagement study group had better mood and quality of life, reduced health costs, and a longer survival time (a 2.7-month advantage) than did control group patients receiving only cancer care (Temel et al. 2010). As one palliative care physician put it, "People usually live longer when they're more comfortable." Other studies have suggested that palliative care prolongs life, but this rigorous, randomized clinical trial was the first to demonstrate that palliative care prolongs survival when delivered concurrently with cancer care.

Palliative care reduces costs. By talking with patients and their families and physicians about the pros and cons of realistic treatment options, palliative care teams help all involved to weigh choices in the context of patient-centered goals and values. A fully informed patient and family who have been given the time and support necessary to come to terms with the patient's illness often (but not always) choose to receive further care in lower-intensity settings. Such care is usually higher quality and often less expensive.

Palliative care is specialized medical care focused on relief from the symptoms, pain, and stress of a serious illness. It is appropriate at any age and at any stage in an illness and can be provided along with curative treatment. The goal is to improve quality of life for both the patient and the family.

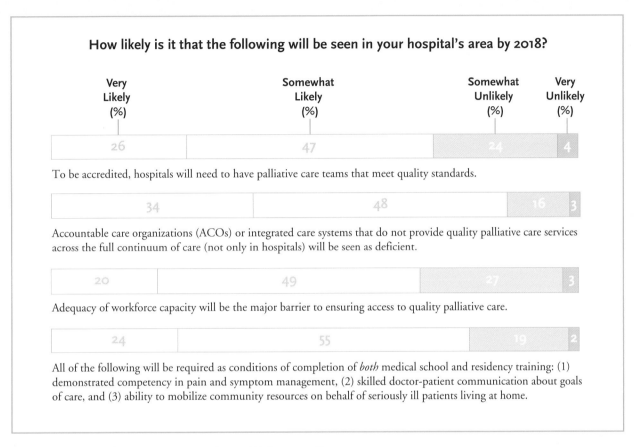

How likely is it that the following will be seen in your hospital's area by 2018?

Very Likely (%)	Somewhat Likely (%)	Somewhat Unlikely (%)	Very Unlikely (%)
26	47	24	4

To be accredited, hospitals will need to have palliative care teams that meet quality standards.

| 34 | 48 | 16 | 3 |

Accountable care organizations (ACOs) or integrated care systems that do not provide quality palliative care services across the full continuum of care (not only in hospitals) will be seen as deficient.

| 20 | 49 | 27 | 3 |

Adequacy of workforce capacity will be the major barrier to ensuring access to quality palliative care.

| 24 | 55 | 19 | 2 |

All of the following will be required as conditions of completion of *both* medical school and residency training: (1) demonstrated competency in pain and symptom management, (2) skilled doctor-patient communication about goals of care, and (3) ability to mobilize community resources on behalf of seriously ill patients living at home.

Note: Percentages in each row may not sum exactly to 100% due to rounding.

What Practitioners Predict

Palliative care will be a regular feature of integrated care. ACOs and other integrated care systems will be expected to provide palliative care services by 2018, according to 82 percent of practitioners; nearly 73 percent expect hospitals will need palliative care teams that meet quality standards in order to be accredited.

Medical training will have new requirements regarding palliative care. There was broad consensus (79 percent of practitioners thought it likely) that by 2018 both medical school and residency training will require the following as conditions of successful completion: (1) demonstrated competency in pain and system management, (2) skill in communication with patients about the goals of care, and (3) ability to mobilize community resources to aid seriously ill patients living at home.

Workforce availability is a concern. Practitioners largely agreed (69 percent thought it likely) that workforce availability will be the major barrier to obtaining quality palliative care by 2018.

The timely involvement of the palliative care team at the point when treatment decisions are being made is key to achieving this outcome. It is through this kind of assistance that palliative care teams across the nation have reduced the costs of care for thousands of patients per hospital per year. A recent study involving eight hospitals and three years of hospital admissions demonstrated an average of $3 million in annual savings for a typical 300-bed community hospital. Costs per day for palliative care patients, both decedents and those who survived to discharge, were dramatically lower than those for patients receiving "usual care" (Morrison et al. 2008). The same results have been achieved at hospitals of all types across the country.

Palliative care also reduces ED visits and rehospitalizations, an important outcome not only for integrated systems such as the Veterans Administration and Kaiser Permanente (Brumley et al. 2007) but for all health systems, given that Medicare ties reimbursement to quality measures such as readmission rates and hospital mortality.

Palliative care improves the value equation. Because palliative care teams both improve quality and reduce costs, they markedly improve the value equation (value = quality ÷ cost) for hospitals, health systems, and the nation as a whole. The positive outcomes of palliative care address the most important challenges facing hospitals today: keeping complex patients and their families safe and satisfied; minimizing unnecessary costs (especially under fixed-payment reimbursement); improving throughput and the ICU and ED "bottlenecks"; keeping specialists busy and happy; minimizing readmissions and hospital mortality; and planning for global budgets,

bundling, and population health management.

Implications for Hospital Leaders

Given these dramatic gains in quality, costs, and survival, the rapid growth of palliative care teams in the United States is not surprising. Although further growth and penetration of these teams will increase their beneficial impact in hospitals, the focus of the future requires integration of palliative care models in the community—nursing homes, assisted living facilities, long-term acute care hospitals, physician office practices, and home care. Community access to palliative care for the seriously ill is the single most important approach to preventing unnecessary and risky hospitalizations among the sickest, most vulnerable, and costliest patients. Effective palliative care management of this group is critical to success under the pay-for-quality and global budgets soon to characterize the US payment and delivery systems.

What steps can healthcare leaders take to strengthen palliative care capacity in their hospitals and communities?

• Conduct a palliative care systems capacity assessment, both in your hospitals and among your community partners.

- Train your workforce in core palliative care competencies.
- Recruit clinical staff with specialist-level palliative care training and board certification.
- Make sure your chief innovation or systems integration officers add development of reliable, standardized, high-quality palliative care to their portfolios.
- Seek Joint Commission (2012) Advanced Certification for Palliative Care in preparation for a probable future accreditation requirement.

We encourage you, as leaders in US healthcare, to consider development or expansion of palliative care programs, not only for your hospital but for your entire healthcare system and your community partners. Answers to the questions most frequently asked by health system leaders are found in the box opposite. ▣

References

Adler, E.D., J.Z. Goldfinger, J. Kalman, M.E. Park, and D.E. Meier. 2009. "Palliative Care in the Treatment of Advanced Heart Failure." *Circulation* 120 (25): 2597–606.

Bakitas, M., K.D. Lyons, M.T. Hegel, S. Balan, F.C. Brokaw, J. Seville, J.G. Hull, Z. Li, T.D. Tosteson, I.R. Byock, and T.A. Ahles. 2009. "Effects of a Palliative Care Intervention on Clinical Outcomes in Patients with Advanced Cancer: The Project ENABLE II Randomized Controlled Trial." *Journal of the American Medical Association* 302 (7): 741–49.

Brumley, R., S. Enguidanos, P. Jamison, R. Seitz, N. Morgenstern, S. Saito, J. McIlwane, K. Hillary, and J. Gonzalez. 2007. "Increased Satisfaction with Care and Lower Costs: Results of a Randomized Trial of In-Home Palliative Care." *Journal of the American Geriatrics Society* 55 (7): 993–1000.

Center to Advance Palliative Care (CAPC). 2012. "Growth of Palliative Care in U.S. Hospitals—2012 Snapshot." Analysis conducted in July. www.capc.org/capc-growth-analysis-snapshot-2011.pdf.

Joint Commission. 2012. "Facts About the Advanced Certification Program for Palliative Care." Published April 2012. www.jointcommission.org/assets/1/18/Palliative_Care.pdf.

Meier, D.E. 2011. "Increased Access to Palliative Care and Hospice: Opportunities to Improve Value in Healthcare." *Milbank Quarterly* 89 (3): 343–80.

Morrison, R.S., J.D. Penrod, J.B. Cassel, M. Caust-Ellenbogen, A. Litke, L. Spragens, and D.E. Meier. 2008. "Cost Savings Associated with US Hospital Palliative Care Consultation Programs." *Archives of Internal Medicine* 168 (16): 1783–90.

National Hospice and Palliative Care Organization (NHPCO). 2012. *NHPCO Facts and Figures: Hospice Care in America*, 2011 edition. www.nhpco.org/files/public/statistics_research/2011_facts_figures.pdf.

Temel, J.S., J.A. Greer, A. Muzikansky, E.R. Gallagher, S. Admane, V.A. Jackson, C.M. Dahlin, C.D. Blinderman, J. Jacobsen, W.F. Pirl, J.A. Billings, and T.J. Lynch. 2010. "Early Palliative Care for Patients with Metastatic Non–Small-Cell Lung Cancer." *New England Journal of Medicine* 363 (8): 733–42.

Wright, A.A., B. Zhang, A. Ray, J.W. Mack, E. Trice, T. Balboni, S.L. Mitchell, V.A. Jackson, S.D. Block, P.K. Maciejewski, and H.G. Prigerson. 2008. "Associations Between End-of-Life Discussions, Patient Mental Health, Medical Care Near Death, and Caregiver Bereavement Adjustment." *Journal of the American Medical Association* 300 (14): 1665–73.

HEALTH INFORMATION EXCHANGES: HELPING HOSPITALS HARNESS THE POWER OF IT

by Carla Smith, John P. Hoyt, FACHE, and Pamela Matthews, RN

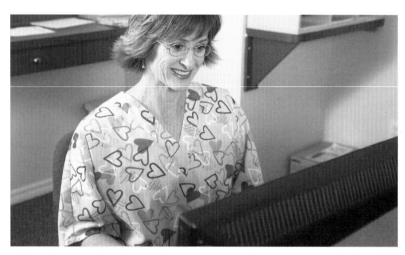

About the Authors

Carla Smith, MA, CNM, is executive vice president of HIMSS, a Chicago-based, not-for-profit organization focused exclusively on providing global leadership for the optimal use of IT and management systems for the betterment of healthcare. As executive vice president, Ms. Smith is responsible for HIMSS's North American focus. She has been involved in the health information and management systems field for 20 years. John P. Hoyt, FACHE, is executive vice president of HIMSS Analytics, which provides data and analytical expertise to support improved decision making by healthcare providers, healthcare IT companies, governments, and consulting firms. Pamela Matthews, RN, MBA, CPHIMS, is HIMSS senior director for regional affairs. All three authors are Fellows of HIMSS.

Healthcare CEOs across the nation are aware of core strategic issues inherent in achieving business success and compliance with three laws: the Healthcare Insurance Portability and Accountability Act of 1996 (HIPAA), the American Recovery and Reinvestment Act of 2009 (ARRA), and the Affordable Care Act of 2010 (ACA). Hospital executives can help their organizations comply with these laws by embracing the strategic power of information technology (IT).

One of the goals of HIPAA was to make the provision of—and payment for—care more cost-effective. To that end, HIPAA called for improving cost-effectiveness by defining financial electronic data interchange (EDI) transaction sets for, among other things, the core processes of eligibility inquiry and response, electronic claim filing and payment, and claim status inquiry and response. (A transaction set is a collection of data that contains all the information required by the receiving system to perform a normal business transaction.) Since 1996, these EDI standards have been further defined and increasingly adopted.

EDI, a well-known construct in healthcare, promises reduced costs and accelerated verification of insurance coverage (eligibility), billing, payment receipt, and claim status. *Health information exchange* (HIE) is a more recent term. Used as a verb ("to exchange health information"), HIE refers to the electronic, secured movement of clinical and business data. Used as a noun, HIE refers to organizations that provide data exchange services to a suite of customers—hospitals, clinical practices, payers, public health agencies, patients, and other health stakeholders.

Both ARRA—specifically, the portion of ARRA known as the HITECH (Health Information Technology for Economic and Clinical Health) Act—and the ACA contain congressional directives to improve the quality, safety, and cost-effectiveness of, and access to, healthcare through the secure, appropriate electronic exchange of heath information. For example, the HITECH Act gives eligible hospitals and professionals financial incentives to demonstrate the ability to securely send and receive health information electronically. To achieve this capability, CEOs can engage in a community-based or state-led HIE, establish their own HIE, or both.

The backbone of EDI and HIE is the ubiquitous use of nationally recognized standards. Standards define how transactions are constructed and transmitted. Ideally, standards eliminate variation in how hospitals, physician practices, private payers, public health officials, and Medicare and Medicaid payers communicate electronically.

Hospitals Slow to Adopt EDI Standards

Since 2009, HIMSS Analytics has collected data on hospitals' adoption and use of HIPAA's EDI standards. The adoption rate is a barometer of the perceived cost/benefit and ease of adopting these standards. Exhibit 5.1 shows the growth in the number of hospitals adopting six EDI transaction sets.

As Exhibit 5.1 shows, the number and percentage of hospitals using the eligibility transaction sets to transmit data directly to payers are extremely low, though increasing. This low use may be due to providers having dedicated connections to their largest payers' eligibility files, through portals or other payer-proprietary applications. Another reason for the low adoption rate is that many providers use a clearinghouse, which receives the nonstandard transaction from the hospital and then formats it into a standard transaction set before forwarding it to the appropriate payer.

Historically, use of a dependable clearinghouse has allowed hospital chief information officers to concentrate on other strategic issues, but reliance on clearinghouses will not suffice in the long run. Adopting eligibility standards frees hospitals to streamline processes and capitalize on operational efficiencies. It also saves hospitals clearinghouse fees, which can be invested in new, strategically impactful IT initiatives.

Adoption of claim status transaction sets has likewise been slow (Exhibit 5.1). Like adoption of eligibility transaction sets, adoption of claim status transaction sets increased from 2009 to 2011 but is far short of where it needs to be to drive the efficiency that providers and the federal government are expecting.

When adopting these standards, hospital executives should integrate information captured and stored by various software applications. Such integration would not only minimize manual and other labor-intensive claim management activities but also enable hospitals to eliminate the per transaction fees of a clearinghouse.

It should come as no surprise that claims submission and payment standards are the ones most used by hospitals (Exhibit 5.1). These standards were among the first to be defined, and they are directly tied to cash flow. Revenue cycle vendors were quick to take advantage of the early standards and deliver products that improved their clients' cash position. In addition, hospitals focused on workflows and operations that yielded faster payments and increased cash on hand. New and emerging payment models, such as accountable care, care coordination, and bundled payments, require continued hospital focus on revenue cycle activities.

Through use of EDI, information technology is emerging as a key tool for new care delivery and payment models. Tracking patient referrals, engaging both staff and nonstaff physicians, sharing clinical data, connecting with business partners, supporting care delivery, and paying for services all require sophisticated use of IT. Hospital resources are stretched as never before, thanks to the Centers for Medicare & Medicaid Services' EHR Incentive Program, its requirement that hospitals and clinical practices be compliant with ICD-10 by October 2014, and new regulations emerging from the ACA. We believe these multiple requirements are major contributors to the low adoption rate of the HIPAA EDI standards. For hospitals to remain operationally viable and sustainable in an era of payment reform, CEOs must shift attention back to these financial standards.

Exhibit 5.1 Nonfederal US Hospitals Adopting EDI Transaction Sets, 2009 and 2011

Transaction Set Type	Percentage (Number) of Hospitals	
	2009 N = 3,748	2011 N = 4,238
Eligibility		
Inquiry (transaction set 270)	11.55% (433)	16.07% (681)
Response (transaction set 271)	10.09% (378)	15.08% (639)
Claim Status		
Inquiry (transaction set 276)	10.81% (405)	15.50% (657)
Response (transaction set 277)	8.99% (337)	11.99% (508)
Claim		
Submission (transaction set 837)	49.81% (1,867)	70.60% (2,992)
Payment (transaction set 835)	29.46% (1,104)	43.18% (1,830)

Source: Data from the Dorenfest Institute for Health Information (www.himss.org/foundation/histdata.asp) and HIMSS Analytics (www.himssanalytics.org/home/index.aspx). Used with permission.

Health information exchange (HIE) is the electronic movement of health-related information among organizations in a secure environment using nationally recognized standards. An HIE organization enables the e-transfer of health-related information that is typically stored at multiple healthcare sites while maintaining the context and integrity of the information being exchanged. Both informal and formal HIEs have been formed across the United States to provide technology, governance, and support for e-exchange of health information.

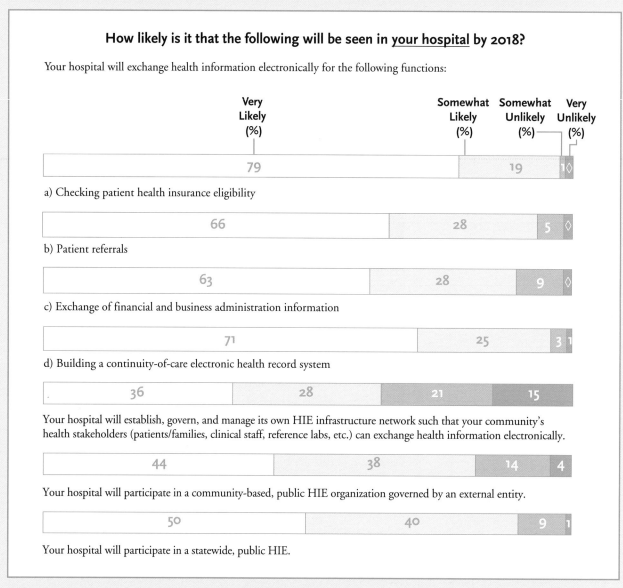

How likely is it that the following will be seen in <u>your hospital</u> by 2018?

Your hospital will exchange health information electronically for the following functions:

	Very Likely (%)	Somewhat Likely (%)	Somewhat Unlikely (%)	Very Unlikely (%)
	79	19	1	◊

a) Checking patient health insurance eligibility

66	28	5	◊	

b) Patient referrals

63	28	9	◊	

c) Exchange of financial and business administration information

71	25	3	1	

d) Building a continuity-of-care electronic health record system

36	28	21	15	

Your hospital will establish, govern, and manage its own HIE infrastructure network such that your community's health stakeholders (patients/families, clinical staff, reference labs, etc.) can exchange health information electronically.

44	38	14	4	

Your hospital will participate in a community-based, public HIE organization governed by an external entity.

50	40	9	1	

Your hospital will participate in a statewide, public HIE.

Note: Percentages in each row may not sum exactly to 100% due to rounding. ◊ Less than 0.5%

Hospital-Owned Versus Nonhospital HIEs

Thanks to emerging payment models and regulatory requirements, deployment of HIE services and organizations continues. Across the nation, hospitals are establishing HIEs to exchange clinical data for care coordination. Additionally, there are regional, community, local, privately owned, and government-owned HIEs. A full 82 percent of *Futurescan* survey respondents indicated their organizations would be likely to participate in a community-based HIE by 2018, and 90 percent would be likely to participate in a state-owned HIE.

A natural outgrowth of hospitals and healthcare systems is the "home-grown" HIE, whose hospital owner manages cost, determines technical strategy and infrastructure, identifies membership, and, most important, controls overall governance of the HIE. Because of this centralized control, the hospital-owned HIE

What Practitioners Predict

Electronic health information exchange will be used for a variety of functions. Practitioners surveyed concurred that by 2018 their hospitals will use electronic HIE for a number of functions. Ninety-eight percent agreed HIE will be used to check patients' insurance eligibility, 96 percent thought it will be used to build a continuity-of-care electronic health record system, more than 94 percent said it will be used for patient referrals, and 91 percent predicted it will be used for exchanging financial and business information.

Hospitals are more likely to use public HIEs than to establish their own. Nearly 90 percent of practitioners thought it likely that by 2018 their hospital would use a statewide, public HIE, while 82 percent thought it likely their hospital would use a community-based, public HIE governed by an external entity. By contrast, 64 percent thought it likely their hospital would establish, govern, and manage its own HIE.

has more flexibility and may launch exchange services more quickly than community-based or state-led HIEs. Sixty-four percent of *Futurescan* survey respondents said their organizations were likely to establish their own HIE infrastructures by 2018—a finding consistent with research by HIMSS and HIMSS Analytics. Hospitals are motivated to launch their own data networks to support new payment and care delivery models.

In contrast with hospital-owned HIEs, state, regional, community, and other types of HIE entities are composed of diverse stakeholder groups. These HIEs provide membership and services through a collaborative stakeholder governance model. Funding can come from multiple sources, such as private parties, government grants, agencies, revenue generation, and participant fee-for-service. The many challenges these HIEs face include gaining stakeholder cooperation, ensuring financial viability, and securing participant trust. Participant trust is particularly sticky because it nearly always involves rethinking of competitive barriers between stakeholders within a community. Navigating the policy and legal issues around data exchange, including privacy and security across and within states, is another significant challenge.

In some sections of the country today, hospital-owned HIEs may connect to several community or regional HIEs as well as to a state-based HIE. In the future, we may also see hospitals and their HIEs connecting to

other independent, private HIEs, such as payer-based exchanges and disease management exchanges. By 2018, we could easily see a national "network of networks" composed of both public and private HIEs, in which providers and other stakeholders connect according to business needs and their financial and clinical operations.

Implications for Hospital Leaders

Hospital-based HIEs may prove to be the linchpin of future data exchange efforts by participating in whatever information exchanges—community, regional, or state-level—satisfy their clinical and financial business needs. By viewing data as a strategic lever, CEOs can position their organizations for long-term sustainability in the new era of payment reform; reduce expenses through avoidance of duplication and unnecessary procedures; and improve the quality of patient care and positive outcomes, thereby increasing patient satisfaction and engagement.

For the myriad patients seeking care from multiple unaffiliated providers; for public health reporting, population health management, and disease surveillance; and for compliance with EDI requirements, hospital executives should ensure their organizations engage with appropriate HIE entities. Given the general perception that hospitals have the most to gain from financial and clinical data exchange, especially in a bundled-payment era, executives should recognize that their hospitals

will be funding the developmental and operating costs of the HIEs.

Thanks to these complexities, hospital executives must ensure long-term sustainability when implementing robust clinical and financial data exchange to achieve business requirements. Planning is critical; hospital HIEs must address these challenges while simultaneously meeting the clinical and business data needs of the hospital or healthcare system.

We recommend that hospital leaders initiate the following steps:

- Ensure that your organization's strategic plan specifically articulates why, how, and under what circumstances the hospital will engage in standards-based EDI and in a hospital-based, community, regional, or state-level HIE.
- Develop an IT strategic plan that addresses federal, state, and payer-based initiatives requiring secure, electronic exchange of clinical and business data.
- Monitor all public and private HIE efforts in your area.
- Participate in efforts that impact your strategic plan.
- Build and invest for the long term, focusing on what you will need in the future, not what you need now. For example, invest in clinical and business intelligence systems, and increase staff competency in this area.
- Invest your time in building relationships and partnerships key to your organization's future success. ⌗

6. MOBILE HEALTHCARE MHEALTH AND THE FUTURE OF HEALTHCARE

by Christopher L. Wasden, EdD

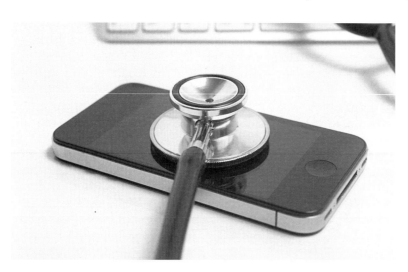

Mobile technology is transforming all industries and markets throughout the world. In the United States cell phones outnumber people, and nearly 50 percent of those are smartphones: small, connected, convergent computers that integrate not only phones but also cameras, TVs, MP3 players, computers, video recorders and players, and even medical devices (Smith 2012). According to Manhattan Research, 62 percent of physicians have a tablet device, double last year's figure (Dolan 2012b).

Like an invincible army, the march of mobile technology advances from industry to industry, conquering and transforming all before it. With each conquest, incumbents that led the old, unconnected world fall as new entrants emerge to deliver better services and experiences to more customers at lower prices. Music, news, books, movies, travel, telecommunications, and banking have already begun a mobile renaissance and are harbingers for how other industries, such as healthcare,

will need to adapt by adopting this disruptive technology.

According to a recent global survey commissioned by PwC and conducted by the Economist Intelligence Unit (2012), healthcare providers and payers believe the widespread adoption of mobile healthcare (mHealth) is inevitable in the near future. Patients in particular expect that mHealth will increase their access to quality care, offer greater convenience, improve engagement and control, and drive down healthcare costs. Doctors believe that mHealth will have as big an impact as the Internet on their relationships with patients and that it will enhance healthcare delivery. It has become clear to healthcare leadership that if organizations don't have a mobile strategy, they haven't got a strategy.

The Mobile Future Is Already Here

Perhaps no healthcare system has demonstrated a stronger commitment to the future of mHealth than the Veterans Health

About the Author

Christopher L. Wasden, EdD, is a managing director and the global healthcare innovation leader at PwC in New York City. At PwC he leads innovation engagements with organizations large and small to help leaders facilitate transformational change that gets innovation into the DNA of the organizational culture, thereby driving growth and success on a sustainable basis. Before joining PwC, Dr. Wasden led nine start-ups, including corporate ventures, venture-financed start-ups, incubators, and family-owned businesses. He is a named inventor on 20 issued patents, and he has written more than 20 reports and papers outlining his philosophy and approach to successful innovation. He holds an EdD degree in human and organizational learning from the George Washington University, an MBA degree from the UCLA Anderson School of Management, and BS and BA degrees in accounting and Asian studies from Brigham Young University.

Administration (VHA). For a decade, the VHA under the leadership of Dr. Adam Darkins has advanced the practice of mHealth, even before it was called that, to improve the quality of care at a fraction of the cost of traditional in-person services. The VHA has conducted extensive studies across thousands of patients and dozens of diseases to demonstrate that mHealth can substantially decrease the costs of chronic disease management, improve drug adherence, decrease readmissions, and enable remote diagnostics and care (Darkins et al. 2008).

Regional healthcare systems have begun to take notice of mHealth's potential and to develop their own solutions for transforming the delivery of care. One regional provider in the southeastern United States delivers remote patient monitoring services to chronic disease patients after discharge without reimbursement from a payer or a fee to the patient (WINKNewsNow 2012). Because Medicare and Medicaid payments do not cover the cost of these patients' emergency visits and hospitalizations and the Centers for Medicare & Medicaid Services will not pay for readmitting these patients, the provider actually saves money by providing these mHealth services for free.

As a result of these successes and mHealth's promising potential, the venture capital community has begun to invest heavily in mHealth applications and devices, committing more than $293 million to this segment in the second quarter of 2012 alone (McCann 2012). Providers such as Partners HealthCare, Cleveland Clinic, and Mayo Clinic have created, and in some instances spun off, mHealth start-ups. Even some smaller regional providers, such as Meridian Health in New Jersey, have followed the lead of these academic medical centers.

Medical device companies are exploring how they can connect their devices to other devices and to health information exchanges and systems. For example, Medtronic recently announced a new remote monitoring technology for its implantable cardiac devices. The *Wall Street Journal* recently profiled how Orthocare Innovations allows patients to use a mobile phone app to program and communicate with its prosthetic devices (Needleman 2012).

It is therefore not surprising that in 2011 the United States spent $660 million on mHealth technology (Dolan 2012a). A recent PwC research report indicated the mHealth market is expected to reach $23 billion by 2017 (PwC and GSMA 2012).

Critical to the growth of this market among providers is the adoption of mobile technologies by physicians and nurses. According to a recent US Bureau of Labor Statistics report, 72 percent of physicians and 71 percent of nurses have smartphones (Hall 2012). This strong penetration of mobile devices among providers accounts for the broad consensus among *Futurescan* survey respondents that mobile devices will be a transformative feature of physician–patient interactions.

Six Factors Affecting mHealth Growth and Adoption

PwC expects the pace of mHealth growth and adoption will continue to accelerate. The following six factors are becoming increasingly important not only in healthcare but across all industries.

mHealth–healthcare integration. Healthcare is becoming more integrated into all aspects of our lives. Retail clinics provide ubiquitous access to care. Schools are adopting healthier menus and incorporating wellness activities. Employers are providing wellness incentives to reward and punish employee behaviors. The pace of mHealth adoption will be determined by how effectively health and wellness activities and services that mesh with consumers' lifestyles are integrated with their devices and applications.

Interoperability. For mHealth devices, apps, and services to provide value, the data and information they generate must be

interoperable among many apps and devices as well as among various personal health records (PHRs), electronic health records (EHRs), and health information exchanges (HIEs). By eliminating redundancies, waste, and errors, interoperability will increase access and quality and reduce costs.

Intelligence. An important but controversial feature of mobile technology is its ability to incorporate intelligence into devices and apps, putting the equivalent of a virtual doctor or nurse in consumers' pockets to guide them through therapy, diagnosis, and wellness activities. This type of intelligence increases patient empowerment, independence, and control. By eliminating the need for direct interaction with professional service providers, intelligence has been a key driver of mobile transformation in other industries.

Social media. A recent PwC report entitled *Social Media "Likes" Healthcare* (PwC 2012) outlined how social media have begun to transform healthcare, a process that will accelerate over time. Social media enable patients to collaborate and share with their peers; allow providers to deliver more useful, timely, and practical guidance and services to patients; and increase the level of support among communities to improve health and wellness.

Better outcomes. One of the most powerful capabilities of mobile devices is their ability to collect data continually on users' location and what they are doing. App developers have begun to harness this capability in novel ways to help patients predict and prevent health-related problems, monitor their compliance with doctors' orders (e.g., prescriptions, diet, activity), review their vital signs, and provide remote patient monitoring services. WellDoc (2011) found that patients monitored

mHealth is a term used for the practice of medicine and public health supported by mobile devices. It most commonly refers to using mobile communication devices, such as mobile phones, tablet computers, and personal digital assistants (PDAs), for health services and information.

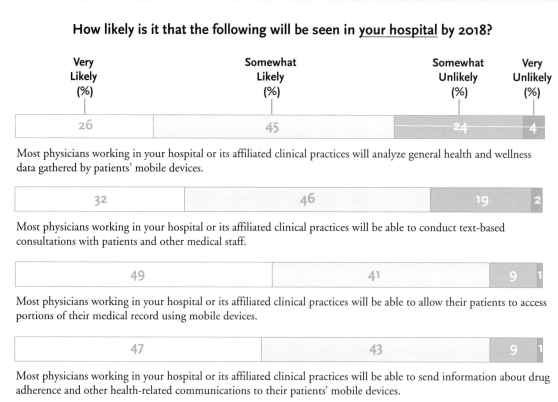

How likely is it that the following will be seen in <u>your hospital</u> by 2018?

Very Likely (%)	Somewhat Likely (%)	Somewhat Unlikely (%)	Very Unlikely (%)
26	45	24	4

Most physicians working in your hospital or its affiliated clinical practices will analyze general health and wellness data gathered by patients' mobile devices.

| 32 | 46 | 19 | 2 |

Most physicians working in your hospital or its affiliated clinical practices will be able to conduct text-based consultations with patients and other medical staff.

| 49 | 41 | 9 | 1 |

Most physicians working in your hospital or its affiliated clinical practices will be able to allow their patients to access portions of their medical record using mobile devices.

| 47 | 43 | 9 | 1 |

Most physicians working in your hospital or its affiliated clinical practices will be able to send information about drug adherence and other health-related communications to their patients' mobile devices.

Note: Percentages in each row may not sum exactly to 100% due to rounding.

What Practitioners Predict

Mobile devices will be a feature of physician and patient interactions. Ninety percent of practitioners predicted that physicians working in their hospital or its affiliated practices will be able to send health-related information to patients and allow patients access to portions of their medical records via their mobile devices by 2018. Seventy-eight percent predicted that physicians will be able to conduct text-based consultations with patients and other medical staff, and 71 percent thought physicians will be able to analyze general health and wellness data gathered from patients' mobile devices.

using its DiabetesManager app, the first FDA-approved mHealth app for diabetes, tended to be more compliant and to find mobile digital tools more effective than older analog tools. Patients who used the app for an average of 12 months reduced their ER visits and hospital stays by 58 percent compared with the previous 12 months.

Patient engagement. Although most patients know what behaviors are healthy and lead to a better quality of life, they don't observe them. A recent study indicated that following seven health recommendations could decrease the risk of death from heart disease by 76 percent (Lloyd-Jones 2012), yet only 1.2 percent of the study's partici-

pants followed all the recommendations, and 92.1 percent followed only one. mHealth has already begun to demonstrate its ability to encourage healthy behaviors and significantly increase patient engagement by providing real-time feedback, intelligent coaching, social interaction, and interoperability integration.

Implications for Hospital Leaders

Mobile experiences in other industries are rapidly and radically changing consumer and patient expectations for healthcare. Consumers ask questions such as "Why can't I use my smartphone to make an appointment with my doctor the way I can book a flight on a travel app? Why can't I order my drugs and pick them up without going to the doctor, seeing that I can buy a book online without going to a bookstore? Why can't I know the price of a healthcare service before I receive it as I can with many online purchases?"

Do you have a strategy that prepares you for the following future patient expectations?

Get ready for on-demand medicine. Patients want services that meet their timing and schedule demands, not those of their doctor. They want to see the doctor's schedule in the palm of their hand and make appointments in real time without waiting. They want copies of their labs, X-rays, and healthcare records on their mobile devices as soon as they are entered into the EHR and made available to the physician. They see no reason for a lag of weeks, days, or even hours. Many virtual retailers, such as Amazon, iTunes, and Kayak, offer instant gratification and response. Consumers expect a similar level of experience when it comes to their healthcare.

Create a new payment model for micromobile services. Just as the music industry had to change its payment model from selling 10 songs on a CD for $15 to selling singles for 99 cents, providers must create a new payment model that offers micromobile services for micropayments. Telefonica Brazil, the major wireless provider in Brazil, just launched a mobile physician call service that allows a cell-phone customer who subscribes for a few *reals* a month to ask a doctor any medical question. In the United States, Teladoc offers something similar. Mobile physician services are also available in Africa, India, and China, where mHealth innovation has moved more quickly than in the United States.

Accept that sunlight (transparency) is the best disinfectant. In nearly every other industry, consumers can use their mobile devices and apps to get detailed information—about the quality of a hotel, the rating and price of a product, or the location and price of a service. Patients want the same in healthcare. They are tired of having to wait two to three months to find out what they owe for services they aren't even sure they received. They know from other industries that transparency is the best cure for waste and inefficiency in a marketplace.

Take two apps and e-mail me in the morning. If an office visit is not required, patients don't want to have to go to the hospital or doctor's office just so a provider can charge a code to get paid. Their time is valuable, and they don't want providers to waste it with frivolous visits. A recent study by the Mayo Clinic revealed that more than 40 percent of healthcare services provided by primary care doctors could be delivered using mobile technologies (Adamson and Bachman 2010). For this reason, the National Health System in the United Kingdom recently advised providers to prescribe an app to avoid a patient office visit if the app could deliver the service (Hammond 2012).

Become continually connected. We can get free Wi-Fi at our local coffee shop or in an airport terminal, but rarely does a hospital or doctor's office offer it. A physician is less likely to share an app, EHR, or X-ray image with a patient on a mobile device if the hospital or office doesn't make it easy to do so. According to the Economist Intelligence Unit (2012), patients expect their providers to be knowledgeable about mHealth apps and to suggest apps the patients should be using. A good starting point would be to provide Wi-Fi within the provider setting to facilitate sharing.

Conclusion

The new mobile paradigm requires a more consumer- and patient-oriented approach to medicine, one that uses mobile technology to increase feedback, change behaviors, and promote engagement and empowerment. By shifting power and control toward the patient, mHealth will change the fundamental nature of the provider–patient relationship.

The changes facilitated by mobile technology will enable providers to increase their productivity and efficiency, provide more frequent, lighter "touches" to more patients, and encourage a better approach to preventive healthcare and wellness. But such changes will also be painful and disruptive, generating powerful, creative tensions that will drive healthcare systems toward the new mobile paradigm. ⑤

References

Adamson, S.C., and J.W. Bachman. 2010. "Pilot Study of Providing Online Care in a Primary Care Setting." *Mayo Clinic Proceedings* 85 (8): 704–710.

Darkins, A., P. Ryan, R. Kobb, L. Foster, E. Edmonson, B. Wakefield, and A.E. Lancaster. 2008. "Care Coordination/Home Telehealth: The Systematic Implementation of Health Informatics, Home Telehealth, and Disease Management to Support the Care of Veteran Patients with Chronic Conditions." *Telemedicine Journal and e-Health* 14 (10): 1118–26.

Dolan, B. 2012a. "Global Mobile Healthcare Market Now Worth $11.8B by 2018." *MobiHealthNews*. Published August 6. http://mobihealthnews.com/18159/global-mobile-health-market-now-worth-11-8b-by-2018/.

————. 2012b. "Physicians Still Use Mobile for Support, Not So Much for Patients Yet." *MobiHealthNews*. Published May 22. http://mobihealthnews.com/17378/physicians-still-use-mobile-for-support-not-so-much-with-patients-yet/.

Economist Intelligence Unit, for PwC. 2012. *Emerging mHealth: Paths for Growth*. Accessed October 17. www.pwc.com/en_GX/gx/healthcare/mhealth/assets/pwc-emerging-mhealth-full.pdf.

Hall, S.D. 2012. "For Nurses, Smartphones at Work Are the Norm." *FierceMobileHealthcare*. Published July 10. www.fiercemobilehealthcare.com/story/nurses-using-smartphones-at-work/2012-07-07.

Hammond, N. 2012. "Patients Told to Use Apps to Check Health." *Marie Claire*. Published February 22. www.marieclaire.co.uk/news/health/535004/patients-told-to-use-apps-to-check-health.html.

Lloyd-Jones, D.M. 2012. "Improving the Cardiovascular Health of the US Population." *Journal of the American Medical Association* 307 (12): 1314–16.

McCann, E. 2012. "VC Funds HIT to the Tune of $293M in Q2." *Healthcare IT News*. Published July 23. www.healthcareitnews.com/news/venture-capital-yields-293m-health-it.

Needleman, S.E. 2012. "New Medical Devices Get Smart." *Wall Street Journal*. Updated August 14. online.wsj.com/article/SB10000872396390444318104577587141033340190.html.

PwC. 2012. *Social Media "Likes" Healthcare: From Marketing to Social Business*. Published April 2012. www.pwc.com/us/en/health-industries/publications/health-care-social-media.jhtml.

PwC and Groupe Spécial Mobile Association (GSMA). 2012. *Touching Lives Through Mobile Health: Assessment of the Global Market Opportunity*. Published February 2012. www.pwc.com/in/en/assets/pdfs/telecom/gsma-pwc_mhealth_report.pdf.

Smith, A. 2012. "Nearly Half of American Adults Are Smartphone Owners." Pew Internet and American Life Project. Published March 1. www.pewinternet.org/Reports/2012/Smartphone-Update-2012.aspx?src=prc-headline.

WellDoc. 2011. "The WellDoc DiabetesManager Cuts Hospitalization and ER Visits in Half." News release issued December 6. www.businesswire.com/news/home/20111206005830/en.

WINKNewsNow. 2012. "New Telemedicine Is Keeping Patients Out of the ER." Story created March 12. www.winknews.com/Local-Florida/2012-03-12/New-telemedicine-is-keeping-patients-out-of-the-ER.

7. GOVERNANCE A TRANSFORMING HEALTHCARE SECTOR REQUIRES BOARDS TO STEP UP THEIR GAME

by Barry S. Bader

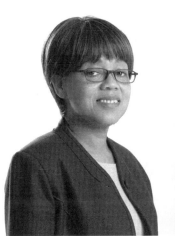

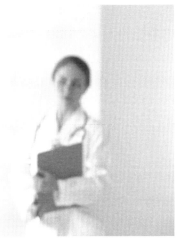

About the Author

Barry S. Bader, president of Bader & Associates in Scottsdale, Arizona, is a consultant, speaker, and retreat facilitator specializing in the governance of hospitals and health systems. He is an advocate for governance effectiveness, accountability, and transparency; streamlined governance structures; board education and active engagement; and a strong partnership between the board and the CEO. Since founding Bader & Associates in 1980, Bader has facilitated board retreats and consulted on governance assessment, restructuring, and redesign initiatives for hospitals, health systems, and other health-related organizations throughout the United States and Canada. Since 1999 he has been one of The Governance Institute's governance advisors and faculty members, and he also has made presentations on governance topics to numerous national and state associations. He has served on the board of trustees of Suburban Hospital, Bethesda, Maryland, and on the Board Quality Committee at Phoenix (Arizona) Children's Hospital.

Several powerful forces have been generating changes in hospital and health system governance for a decade and more, and are likely to intensify in coming years.

Higher Expectations

Higher expectations for corporate accountability and director professionalism are requiring boards to be more independent, accountable, and transparent and to follow best practices to optimize their effectiveness.

The Sarbanes–Oxley Act of 2002 (SOX) set new expectations for director independence, audit and compliance oversight, competency-based boards, and application of best practices. Governance experts urge going beyond formal structures and practices to create a culture of candor and engagement in which informed boards are not afraid to question management about corporate strategy, operating performance, and ethical conduct (Sonnenfeld 2002; Prybil 2008). Although largely exempt from SOX, the not-for-profit sector has embraced its spirit; leading not-for-profit associations have offered best-practice recommendations (Independent Sector 2007; AHA Center for Healthcare Governance 2009; Alliance for Advancing Nonprofit Health Care 2011; Prybil et al. 2012).

Economic Pressures

Economic pressures are driving health systems to optimize their performance and ensure that their governance structure facilitates system-wide synergies and economies of size and scale. As payers constrain payments and link reimbursement to quality outcomes, multiunit systems have found that optimizing performance requires tighter coordination, centralization, shared services, and standardization across operating units.

To prevent subsidiary boards from acting as the "tail wagging the dog" and slowing needed improvements, some health systems have restructured by consolidating or eliminating local boards, changing their roles to advisory ones, and replacing representational formulas for populating parent boards with competency-based processes that choose directors who put the interests of the entire system before parochial concerns. At the same time, multiunit systems need new mechanisms to maintain community connectedness and effective oversight of local facilities without local fiduciary boards.

Physician–Hospital Integration

The increasing economic alignment of hospitals and physicians requires that boards recognize the importance

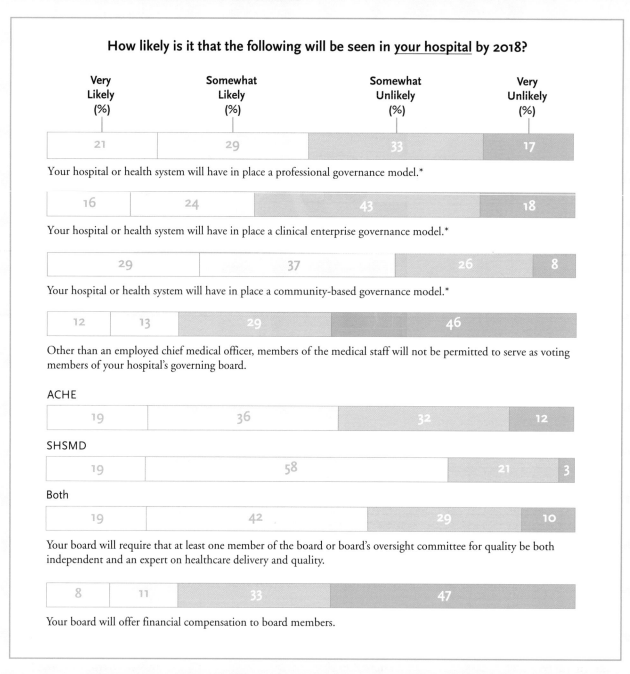

How likely is it that the following will be seen in <u>your hospital</u> by 2018?

Very Likely (%)	Somewhat Likely (%)	Somewhat Unlikely (%)	Very Unlikely (%)
21	29	33	17

Your hospital or health system will have in place a professional governance model.*

16	24	43	18

Your hospital or health system will have in place a clinical enterprise governance model.*

29	37	26	8

Your hospital or health system will have in place a community-based governance model.*

12	13	29	46

Other than an employed chief medical officer, members of the medical staff will not be permitted to serve as voting members of your hospital's governing board.

ACHE

19	36	32	12

SHSMD

19	58	21	3

Both

19	42	29	10

Your board will require that at least one member of the board or board's oversight committee for quality be both independent and an expert on healthcare delivery and quality.

8	11	33	47

Your board will offer financial compensation to board members.

Note: Percentages in each row may not sum exactly to 100% due to rounding.   *See accompanying article for description.

of physician engagement and physician leadership development to the success of an integrated delivery system. The transformation of hospitals from a doctor's workshop into a team workspace is challenging and has governance implications. For example, although physician trustees bring expertise and perspectives on patient care, boards increasingly find that physicians have potential conflicts of interest as either employees or competitors of the hospital.

Challenges to Tax-Exempt Status

Over the past decade, not-for-profit hospitals and health systems have faced a series of challenges to their tax-exempt status from municipal governments, state legislatures and courts, state attorneys general, Congress, and the Internal Revenue Service (IRS). Not-for-profit hospitals have been challenged on their levels of charity care and other community benefits, executive

Practitioners are divided about governance models. A majority (nearly 66 percent) of practitioners thought it likely that by 2018 their hospitals will have a community-based governance model, which places the highest priority on community connectedness and optimizes opportunities for stakeholder input. In this model, 12 to 25 board members, in addition to the CEO, reflect the diversity of stakeholders in the communities served.

Practitioners were evenly split on whether their hospitals will have a professional governance model, which features a lean structure and a board composed of individuals with the necessary competencies who give board work the same priority as service on a corporate board.

Nearly 40 percent of practitioners predicted their hospitals will have a clinical enterprise governance model, with a small parent board and a clinical enterprise board accountable to the parent board and consisting of senior executives and aligned physicians responsible for organizational decision making, leadership, and implementation.

Medical staff members will be voting members of governing boards. Three-quarters of practitioners thought it unlikely that chief medical officers will be the only medical staff serving as voting members of their hospitals' governing boards by 2018.

Views are mixed on whether quality experts will be required for boards. A majority of practitioners (61 percent) thought their hospital boards will be required to have at least one independent expert on healthcare delivery and quality (much as the Sarbanes–Oxley Act requires a financial expert on corporate audit committees) by 2018.

Board members are unlikely to be compensated. Most of the practitioners surveyed (more than 80 percent) thought it somewhat or very unlikely that members of their hospitals' boards will be compensated financially by 2018.

compensation practices, perks for board members, and oversight of corporate compliance. The IRS has expanded disclosure requirements on the Form 990 in such areas as board conflicts of interest, executive compensation, and community benefit. The Affordable Care Act requires regular community health assessments. As a result, boards are embracing stronger public accountability and oversight responsibilities for their organizations' community benefit, stewardship of resources, and ethical conduct.

Key Assumptions

The most certain forecast about the future in healthcare is that uncertainty is likely to prevail for some time. Several trends related to governance are likely to emerge under most healthcare reform scenarios:

- Pressures for professionalism in governance—accountable, independent, and effective boards—will continue and intensify.

- The need to transform healthcare organizations to optimize system performance and generate cost savings will accelerate, driven by tightening reimbursements and value-based payments. The changes will require boards to be visionary, strategic, and prepared to lead amid uncertainty and industry-wide change.
- Care systems' financial objectives cannot be achieved without high-level attention to improving quality and value and addressing community health and health disparities.
- The transformation of hospitals from a fee-for-service, acute care orientation to a value-driven, patient- and population-centered care delivery system will entail both opportunity and increased risk. Boards will need to incorporate enterprise risk management methods into their work, including assessment and oversight of business and financial risks, compliance and regulatory risks,

reputational risks, and information security risks.

Implications for Hospital and Health System Leaders

Based on these assumptions, leaders of hospitals and health systems may need to consider these major governance implications:

Boards will need to formally revisit their governance roles, structures, and practices to ensure they are positioned to provide the leadership and oversight needed by integrated, accountable care systems. Most current hospital and health system governance structures and practices were forged when the delivery system was hospital-centric, dominated by freestanding, community-based acute care facilities and, in recent years, by consolidation of hospitals into health systems. Although there is wide variation in board cultures and effectiveness, many boards have similar "DNA" passed down from hospital ancestors. They draw most trustees locally from the community's "elite" establishment, favoring individuals with business and finance backgrounds. Viewing board service as a volunteer position can lead to low expectations for participation, large boards to make up for poor attendance, a permissive attitude toward conflicts of interest, overly powerful cliques, and letting philanthropy outweigh problematic conduct.

Community boards so cherish local autonomy that they may not objectively evaluate strategic alliance and merger opportunities. The medical staff president and other officers may serve as ex officio representatives of a medical staff that is viewed not as a care partner, but warily as a semiautonomous entity with a self-centered economic agenda.

Integrated and accountable care systems will require recognizing the presence of these strands of hospital DNA and replacing them with new approaches.

As hospitals transform into care systems, their hospital-based governance models will need to evolve to reflect the desired essential characteristics of their systems. Currently, forward-thinking systems are gravitating toward one of three governance models (Exhibit 7.1) or "cross-pollinating" key attributes from each into a hybrid model. The *Futurescan* survey results indicate how leaders see governance evolving in the future:

- A *professional governance model* was seen as likely by half the respondents. This model is designed for health systems that see themselves as a "health company" that, although not-for-profit in motive, embodies the culture of a high-performing, customer-focused corporate enterprise. Governance will be a professional commitment, with higher performance expectations than for the typical volunteer board. A lean-sized parent board of independent directors plus the CEO will have formal authority, although advisory bodies may be maintained or created.
- Forty percent of respondents see a *clinical enterprise governance model* emerging by 2018, as the organization becomes a "physician-driven and professionally managed" patient care delivery system. It will usually feature dual boards: a corporate parent or foundation board with independent members, ultimate authority, and responsibility for independent oversight and high-level goal setting; and an empowered and active "clinical enterprise" board of senior executives and senior physician and nursing leaders accountable to the parent board.
- An *enhanced community-based governance model* will remain the most common model for hospitals that see themselves as closely connected to their community. The parent board will be drawn mainly from the communities served but will adopt various best practices to make board recruitment more objective, meetings more strategic, and oversight more rigorous. The board will place a high priority on strategic thinking, quality leadership, community benefit, and health disparities issues as well as on philanthropy.

Recognized "best" practices that today are aspirational will become the baseline in an era of high expectations. These best practices include the following:

- The CEO wants an informed and engaged board and actively supports its work.
- Board work is focused on high-level, future-oriented strategy and policy, not operational matters.
- The board chair is chosen for his or her leadership skills, based on objective competencies.
- New board members are recruited and elected using competency-based criteria.
- The board promotes a culture of accountability, trust, collaboration, candor, engagement, continuous learning, and ethical conduct.
- New-member orientation and continuing education are ongoing.
- A streamlined size and committee structure facilitate efficient oversight and nimble decision making.
- Dashboards and balanced scorecard–style reports clearly highlight performance successes and variations for board oversight.
- The board engages in a regular self-assessment process and uses the results to drive continuous improvement.
- The performance of individual trustees is evaluated, and the results are used to provide helpful feedback and to base reelection on demonstrated effectiveness.
- In multiorganizational systems that retain local or subsidiary boards, there is clear delineation of the authority and value-added roles of the parent and subsidiary bodies, including whether the latter have governing or advisory power.

Boards will need to adopt leadership tools that are suited to transforming organizations in an uncertain economic environment. These tools include the following:

- Elevating to a strategic level the issues and questions addressed at a governance and leadership level in the organization
- Adopting scenario-based strategic planning methods so the board can examine various "what if" alternatives and be better prepared for the twists and turns of an uncertain environment
- Using inquiry-oriented (as opposed to advocacy-driven) decision-making processes for

selected decisions with large, long-term ramifications (Garvin and Roberto 2001)

- Using "bifocal metrics" to assess both current-year performance and progress toward the organization's vision as an accountable care system or part of one
- Using enterprise risk management techniques to assess the many types of risk—financial, strategic, regulatory, and reputational—that exist in a changing environment

Boards will need to strengthen succession planning to elect trustees with the right professional backgrounds and—just as important—the right "boardroom skills" to govern a care system. Key actions include the following:

- Giving careful thought to the subject area backgrounds and professional skills effective governance will require, such as finance, quality, compliance, and executive leadership of a complex enterprise
- Ensuring that the board's makeup includes at least one independent expert in each of the board's core fiduciary responsibilities
- Ensuring that the board also includes competencies appropriate to a broadened care system vision, such as backgrounds in cultural transformation, population and community health, patient engagement, enterprise risk management, and information technology
- Identifying individuals who have both prior board experience and a "governance temperament"—that is, such boardroom skills as strategic and visionary thinking, systems thinking, critical questioning and analysis, and the ability to lead and inspire as part of a team

These expectations may be unreachable if boards continue to rely solely on local recruitment. Boards will need to become more comfortable identifying potential

Exhibit 7.1 Three Emerging Care System Governance Models

Professional Governance

Clinical Enterprise Governance

Enhanced Community-based Governance

trustees from outside their service areas who bring the required competencies, independence, and diversity and who can work effectively with locally based trustees.

Boards will elevate quality from primarily oversight to a strategic priority that is integral to delivery system redesign and cultural transformation. Several studies in recent years have identified specific governance practices that are associated with high-performing, higher-quality healthcare organizations (Ashish and Epstein 2010; Vaughn et al. 2006; Jiang et al. 2008). These include making quality a priority agenda item for substantive discussion at all or most board meetings, spending at least 20 percent of time discussing quality performance, having a board quality subcommittee, reviewing a dashboard regularly, including quality objectives in the CEO's performance evaluation, and participating with medical staff leaders in establishing quality and patient safety goals. In addition, future governance leaders should consider these actions:

- Requiring that the board include at least one independent expert in medical quality; also, considering backgrounds in nursing, public health, and industrial quality assurance
- Adopting performance metrics beyond acute care to reflect the care system's broader mission and accountability for patient outcomes in all settings, improved health status, adoption of healthy behaviors, reduced absenteeism/workplace injuries, elimination of unjustified variations in care, and so forth
- Seeking the advice of independent quality auditors, chosen by and accountable to the board, much as boards today get an unvarnished financial assessment from an outside auditor

Boards will devote increased attention to their public accountability for community benefit, responsible stewardship of resources, and ethical conduct. In 2007, the American Hospital Association recommended policies and guidelines to promote accountability and transparency of billing, financial assistance policies, and collection practices, as well as to promote community health (AHA 2007). The following are actions boards should consider:

- Advocating for clear and consistent regulatory requirements for tax exemption at a federal, state, and local level
- Educating board members on how to interpret and use community health assessments and strategic plans for implementation
- Understanding leverage points and strategies for engaging patients and changing individual behaviors
- Building greater capacity for collaboration with partners with compatible goals and capabilities
- Establishing a board-level committee to give high priority and leadership to community benefit and community health improvement

The role of physician members of the governing board will change to reflect the need for director independence and competence in governance skills. New methods other than board seats will emerge to fully engage physicians in organizational leadership and direction setting, particularly affecting patient care (Bader 2011). The following are among the actions to consider:

- Choosing physician board members using the same process and competency-based criteria as for all directors, and eliminating any ex officio voting seats for medical staff officers (barring all active medical staff from serving on the board is unlikely, however)
- Cocreating, based on a shared vision, a clinical leadership infrastructure, including such mechanisms as a medical group board that reports to the hos-

pital board, boards of clinically integrated physician–hospital organizations and joint-venture clinical institutes, physician members of the board's quality committee, clinical service lines comanaged by a nurse and a physician executive, and accountable physician leaders for major clinical departments

Conclusion

Just as hospitals moving from fee-for-service reimbursement to value-based payments have one foot in the past and one in the future, so will boards find practices hardwired from their past that may suboptimize future performance. These must change. Boards need to ensure they have a robust capacity for regular self-examination and a willingness to change ahead of a major crisis so they can lead their organizations as the industry around them transforms. 🖾

References

Alliance for Advancing Nonprofit Health Care. 2011. *Great Governance: A Practical Guide for Busy Board Leaders and Executives of Nonprofit Health Care Organizations*. Approved August 9. www.nonprofithealthcare.org/uploads/Alliance-GreatGovernanceGuide.pdf.

American Hospital Association (AHA). 2007. *Community Accountability and Transparency*. Published in November. www.aha.org/content/00-10/07accountability.pdf.

American Hospital Association's Center for Healthcare Governance and Health Research & Educational Trust. 2009. *Competency-Based Governance: A Foundation for Board and Organizational Effectiveness*. Published in February. www.americangovernance.com/americangovernance/BRP/files/brp-2009.pdf.

Ashish, J., and A. Epstein. 2010. "Hospital Governance and the Quality of Care." *Health Affairs* 29 (1): 182–87.

Bader, B. 2011. "Physicians on Hospital Boards: Time for New Approaches." *American Hospital Association's Great Boards*. Published February 1. www.greatboards.org/newsletter/2011/GreatBoards-reprint-2011-Physicians-on-Hospital-Boards.pdf.

Garvin, D.A., and M.A. Roberto. 2001. "What You Don't Know About Making Decisions." *Harvard Business Review* 79 (8): 108–16, 161.

Independent Sector, Panel on the Nonprofit Sector. 2007. *Principles for Good Governance and Ethical Practice: A Guide for Charities and Foundations*. Published in October. www.independentsector.org/uploads/Accountability_Documents/Principles_for_Good_Governance_and_Ethical_Practice.pdf.

Jiang, H.J., C. Lockee, K. Bass, and I. Fraser. 2008. "Board Engagement in Quality: Findings of a Survey of Hospital and System Leaders." *Journal of Healthcare Management* 53 (2): 121–34.

Prybil, L. 2008. "What's Your Board's Culture?" *Trustee* 61 (6): 16–18, 23.

Prybil, L., S. Levey, R. Killian, D. Fardo, R. Chait, D. Bardach, and W. Roach. 2012. *Governance in Large Nonprofit Health Systems: Current Profile and Emerging Patterns*. Commonwealth Center for Governance Studies, Inc. Published in August. www.americangovernance.com/americangovernance/files/governance-booklet.pdf.

Sonnenfeld, J.A. 2002. "What Makes Great Boards Great." *Harvard Business Review* 80 (9): 106–13.

Vaughn, T., M. Koepke, E. Kroch, W. Lehrman, S. Sinha, and S. Levey. 2006. "Engagement of Leadership in Quality Improvement Initiatives: Executive Quality Improvement Survey Results." *Journal of Patient Safety* 2 (1): 2–9.

THE FUTURE OF BALDRIGE-BASED PERFORMANCE EXCELLENCE

by Harry S. Hertz, PhD, HFACHE

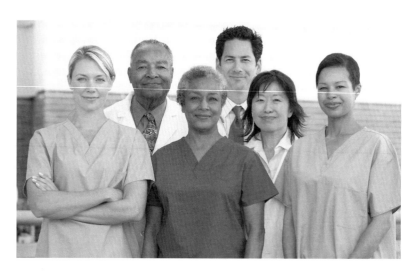

About the Author

Harry S. Hertz, PhD, is director of the Baldrige Performance Excellence Program of the National Institute of Standards and Technology of the US Department of Commerce. Before becoming program director in 1996, he served as the program's deputy director from 1992 to 1996. Dr. Hertz has been with the National Institute of Standards and Technology since 1973, originally as a research chemist, then in a series of management positions, including director of the Chemical Science and Technology Laboratory. He has made presentations to a wide variety of audiences on the Malcolm Baldrige National Quality Award, its criteria for measuring performance excellence, and healthcare and education quality improvement. Dr. Hertz is the author or coauthor of more than 50 publications and holds one patent. He has a BS in chemistry from the Polytechnic Institute of Brooklyn and a PhD from MIT. He is an Honorary Fellow of the American College of Healthcare Executives.

In 1987, when the Malcolm Baldrige National Quality Improvement Act was signed into law by President Ronald Reagan, quality was assumed to be a subject that process and statistics professionals worried about. The quality challenge was taken strictly to be one of improving US manufactured goods to match the much better quality of global competitors, such as Japan and Germany. Very few people perceived a quality challenge in healthcare. Indeed, it was the quality challenge in manufactured goods that led to the creation of the Baldrige Award as a Presidential award to recognize role-model companies willing to share their best practices with other US companies.

The Baldrige Program was also assigned responsibility for developing criteria any business could use to self-assess and improve its quality. From the start, many more companies used the Baldrige Criteria to improve than applied for the Baldrige Award.

In the mid-1990s, with the Baldrige Program enjoying consid-

erable success in the business community, that community approached the program about bringing the benefits of Baldrige to healthcare and education. Criteria specific to healthcare were developed, and a pilot program was conducted in 1995. The pilot was a great success, and a movement began to create an official healthcare category for the Baldrige Award. The category was established through a change in the law in 1998.

Over time, the focus of the Baldrige Program has evolved, as have the Criteria. Today, the Health Care Criteria for Performance Excellence (Baldrige Performance Excellence Program 2011) are widely used and viewed as a road map for organizational performance excellence.

Performance excellence is defined as an integrated approach to organizational performance management that results in

- delivery of ever-improving value to patients, other customers, and stakeholders, contributing to

improved healthcare quality and organizational sustainability;
- improvement of overall organizational effectiveness and capabilities; and
- organizational and personal learning.

This definition is realized through questions presented in the seven interrelated Baldrige Criteria categories illustrated in Exhibit 8.1. These questions relate to both the individual categories and the linkages (indicated by arrows) among

Exhibit 8.1 Health Care Criteria Framework: A Systems Perspective

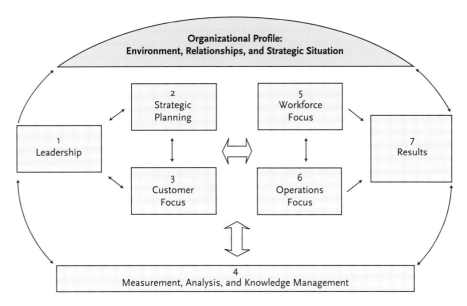

Source: Baldrige Performance Excellence Program.

the category building blocks. These linkages help organizations think holistically about everything that is important to success and sustainability, rather than practicing siloed thinking.

For example, in many organizations strategic planning (category 2) is the domain of senior executives, and workforce focus (category 5) is the domain of human resources departments, with little coordination between the two and even less coordination among executives, managers, and human resources departments on the hiring and development needs associated with building future organizational core competencies (part of strategic planning, category 2). The Criteria ask questions that relate strategic planning to workforce focus needs and future core competencies. The Criteria thus promote a view of the organization as a "whole organism" rather than a collection of "body parts."

Why Use Baldrige?

This question is commonly asked in the context of other tools and methods being used to ensure quality.

Baldrige is a holistic approach. Baldrige addresses everything that is important to a successful healthcare provider—from strategy development to healthcare outcomes, patient satisfaction, and financial results. An assessment against the Criteria yields strengths to build on and opportunities for improvement, all aimed at taking the organization to a higher level of performance. Techniques such as Six Sigma and Lean complement a Baldrige assessment, by providing methods for improving operational performance once areas of focus have been identified. Accreditation sets the acceptable level of performance, while Baldrige identifies steps to achieve even higher performance. The feedback from accreditation is deficiencies; the feedback from Baldrige is strengths and opportunities.

Baldrige is aligned with IOM and IHI. Baldrige helps organizations address the Institute of Medicine's Six Aims for Improvement in providing safe, effective, patient-centered, timely, efficient, and equitable healthcare (Committee on Quality of Health Care in America 2001).

It guides organizations in achieving the Institute for Healthcare Improvement's Triple Aim of improving the patient experience (including quality and satisfaction), improving the health of populations, and reducing the per capita cost of care (2007).

Baldrige hospitals outperform their peers. A recent Thomson Reuters study (Foster and Chenoweth 2011) found substantial agreement between the results of the Baldrige process and Thomson Reuters' data-based 100 Top Hospitals award:

- Hospitals that have been Baldrige award recipients are significantly more likely than their peers to win a 100 Top Hospitals national award.
- Baldrige hospitals were significantly more likely than their peers to display faster five-year performance improvement.
- As a group, Baldrige hospitals were about 83 percent more likely than non-Baldrige hospitals to be awarded a 100 Top Hospitals national award for

The Baldrige Performance Excellence Program is the nation's public–private partnership dedicated to helping all organizations improve their performance and competitiveness. The Baldrige Program disseminates evaluation criteria and manages the Malcolm Baldrige National Quality Award. The criteria and the award process have seen a steady increase in the healthcare sector over the past decade.

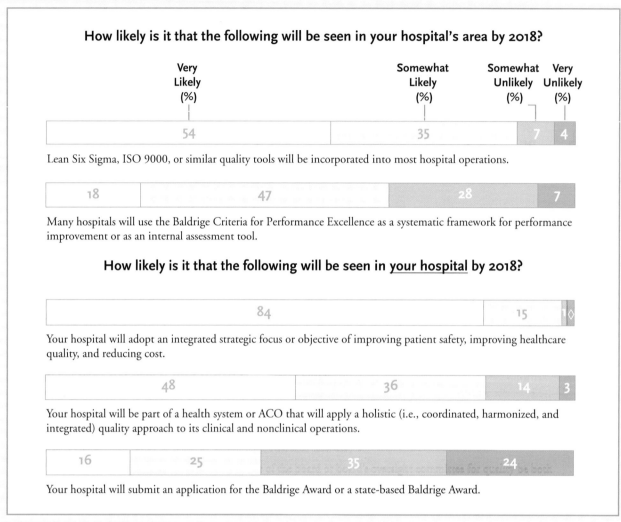

Note: Percentages in each row may not sum exactly to 100% due to rounding.   ◊ Less than 0.5%

What Practitioners Predict

Quality tools will be part of most hospital operations. Practitioners concurred that quality tools such as Lean Six Sigma and ISO 9000 will be integrated into hospital operations, with 89 percent saying this was somewhat or very likely by 2018. A majority (more than 65 percent) predicted that many hospitals will use the Baldrige Criteria as a systematic framework for performance improvement or as an internal assessment tool.

Hospitals will adopt integrated strategies for safety, quality, and cost reduction. Almost all practitioners surveyed (99 percent) believed their hospitals will adopt an integrated strategic focus on improving patient safety and healthcare quality and reducing cost by 2018. Eighty-four percent predicted their hospital will be part of a health system or ACO that will apply a holistic quality approach to its clinical and nonclinical operations.

Some hospitals will apply for a Baldrige award. Forty-one percent of practitioners predicted their hospitals will submit an application for a national or state-based Baldrige award by 2018.

excellence in balanced organization-wide performance.

- Baldrige hospitals outperformed non-Baldrige hospitals on nearly all of the individual measures of performance used in the 100 Top Hospitals composite score.

Why use Baldrige? Because it provides a mechanism for simultaneously focusing on cost, safety, patient care and health outcomes, operational effectiveness, and the short and long term.

Trends in Baldrige Use

The healthcare community has made growing use of the Baldrige Criteria, as evidenced by an increase in downloads of the Health Care Criteria from the Baldrige website (Exhibit 8.2) and applications for the Baldrige Award (Exhibit 8.3). Downloads have increased from just under 300,000 in 2002 to more than 600,000 in 2011. Healthcare award applications have risen from under 20 percent of total applications to more than 50 percent. Based on the *Futurescan* survey results indicating that nearly 66 percent of respondents will be using Baldrige Criteria

and 41 percent will be applying for the national Baldrige award or a Baldrige-based state award by 2018, these trends should not only continue but accelerate.

Perhaps the most satisfying trend is the improvement in performance among healthcare organizations that apply for the Baldrige Award. Exhibit 8.4a shows the disparity in performance between healthcare organizations and for-profit service businesses in 1995. Exhibit 8.4b shows how this disparity has disappeared over time; the performance of leading healthcare organizations now parallels that of leading service companies.

Implications for Hospital Leaders

The Baldrige Criteria continue to evolve. Baldrige intends the Criteria always to reflect the leading edge of validated management practice. Knowing that the most significant changes in the 2013–2014 Criteria will be in the areas of work systems (how organizations accomplish their work), innovation, and social media use, I speculate here on some significant implications for hospital

leaders of these and future Criteria updates.

Focus on business model innovation. Hospital leaders appreciate the constant impact of technological innovation on the delivery of healthcare and on the financial challenges they face. Business model innovation is a second type of innovation that will be a constant focus of strategic consideration over the next five to ten years. Shifts to integrated delivery systems, a focus on population health, and responsibility for covered lives all will challenge hospital leaders to explore and develop new business models.

This systemic change is not unique to healthcare. In the recent *2012 Global CEO Study* (IBM 2012), which surveyed 1,700 leaders in 64 countries and a broad cross section of business and public sectors, a key finding was that CEOs need to amplify innovations with partnerships. The report stated that CEOs need to break from the status quo and make use of external catalysts to cause disruptive thinking. In healthcare, the initial set of external catalysts is a product of the changing environment. How will

Exhibit 8.2 Downloads of the Baldrige Health Care Criteria, 2002 to 2011

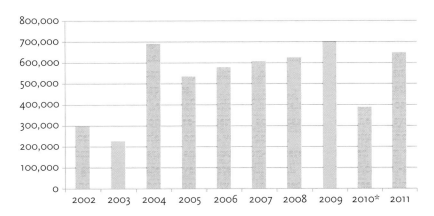

*Beginning in 2009, the Criteria have been produced every two years. The 2010 figure represents downloads in the second year of availability of the 2009–2010 Criteria.

Source: Data from Baldrige Performance Excellence Program.

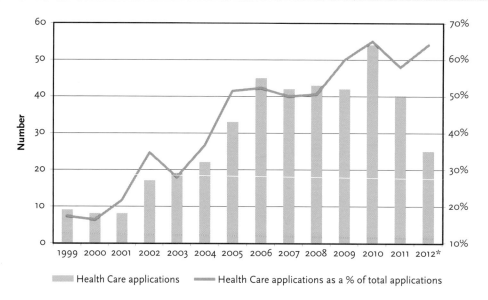

Health Care applications

Health Care applications as a % of total applications

*In 2012, Baldrige Award eligibility rules changed to limit applications to organizations that had received the top award from an Alliance for Performance Excellence state- or sector-based program.

Source: Data from Baldrige Performance Excellence Program.

hospital senior leaders take control of the environment to drive the next generation of external catalysts?

Engage with social media. A McKinsey study of 4,200 global executives (Bughin, Byers, and Chui 2011) reported that more than 50 percent of respondents used social networking, and more than 40 percent used blogs. In the *2012 Global CEO Study* (IBM 2012), CEOs indicated that collaboration was the number one trait they seek in their employees, with 75 percent calling it critical and social media providing a key opportunity.

Four distinct areas stand out in the growing use of social media. The first is use of social media as a vehicle for communicating with staff. Internal wikis allow knowledge sharing and knowledge building, and internal CEO blogging allows two-way communication that breaks down the organizational hierarchy and eliminates distance. The second

area is coordination with partners, suppliers, and collaborators. Social media permit more efficient total healthcare value chain operation and appropriate knowledge sharing.

The third area is communication with patients and customers by means of Facebook, Twitter, web-based healthcare information, blogs, and other mass outreach activities, as well as communicating with individual customers about their complaints and ideas. Finally, social media provide a potential gold mine of external data and information about customer perceptions, desires, and evaluations of your services. Hospital leaders should be using these data for operational and strategic change.

Build healthy communities. The concept of healthy communities has two components. The first deals with the health status of the people in the community—that is, population health—and the realization that integrated healthcare delivery

means hospital leaders will become more involved in the health of the patient population outside the hospital's four walls.

The second component deals with the vitality of the community as a whole and involves healthcare leaders working with business, education, and community leaders to build a healthy, vibrant, and economically sustainable community. The focus on healthy communities is not only an anticipated future strategic challenge; it is also the right business decision. Numerous studies indicate that consumers will increasingly consider social responsibility in their spending decisions (see, for example, Frighetto 2012), so a focus on a healthy community will be a competitive advantage. The Baldrige Criteria are likely to be used as a framework for assessing and guiding strategic improvements in community performance.

Think and act strategically. Managing a healthcare enterprise

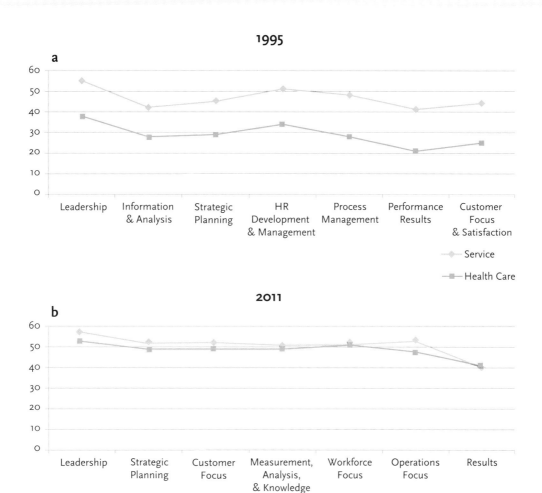

Source: Data from Baldrige Performance Excellence Program.

will become increasingly complex because of changes in regulation, consolidation, payment and reimbursement systems, uncertain economic conditions, and integrated delivery systems. To address these changes and the inherent uncertainty associated with them, leaders will have to be able to adjust strategy quickly and execute changes rapidly. This complexity will require strategic agility and simplicity in communication and execution to deal with ongoing change. Dealing with uncertainty by avoiding strategic planning will likely be fatal for an institution. Starting in 2013, the Baldrige Criteria will include a focus on dealing with strategy in uncertain times. 🄵🅂

References

Baldrige Performance Excellence Program. 2011. *2011–2012 Health Care Criteria for Performance Excellence.* Accessed October 9, 2012. www.nist.gov/baldrige/publications/upload/2011_2012_Health_Care_Criteria.pdf.

Bughin, J., A.H. Byers, and M. Chui. 2011. "How Social Technologies Are Extending the Organization." *McKinsey Quarterly.* Published November 2011. www.mckinseyquarterly.com/How_social_technologies_are_extending_the_organization_2888.

Committee on Quality of Health Care in America, Institute of Medicine. 2001. *Crossing the Quality Chasm: A New Health System for the 21st Century.* Released March 1. www.iom.edu/Reports/2001/Crossing-the-Quality-Chasm-A-New-Health-System-for-the-21st-Century.aspx.

Foster, D.A., and J. Chenoweth. 2011. *Comparison of Baldrige Award Applicants and Recipients with Peer Hospitals on a National Balanced Scorecard.* Published October 2011. www.nist.gov/baldrige/upload/baldrige-hospital-research-paper.pdf.

Frighetto, J. 2012. "Nielsen Identifies Attributes of the Global, Socially-Conscious Consumer." News release published March 27. www.nielsen.com/us/en/insights/press-room/2012/nielsen-identifies-attributes-of-the-global--socially-conscious-.html.

IBM Corporation. 2012. *2012 Global CEO Study.* Accessed September 4. www.ibm.com/ceostudy2012.

Institute for Healthcare Improvement. 2007. "IHI Triple Aim Initiative." Accessed September 4, 2012. www.ihi.org/offerings/initiatives/tripleaim/pages/default.aspx.